This book provides a detailed overview of the function of the nervous system in fever and its role in antipyresis. The volume opens with an introductory account of fever, its physiology and adaptive role, and explains the mechanisms of thermoregulation. Sufficient information about bacterial pyrogens, 'endogenous' pyrogenic cytokines, body temperature regulation and survival value of fever and its ubiquity is given to enable readers to follow the CNS involvement. The book should enable graduate students and researchers in neuroscience and other disciplines to understand the impact of their studies in the overall processes of fever. It will also be of benefit to pharmacologists studying antipyretics and the CNS function of these drugs. Academic clinicians will find this a more comprehensive overview of fever than other available texts. Finally, the author challenges some well-established dogmas in this area and sets an agenda for future research.

FEVER AND ANTIPYRESIS

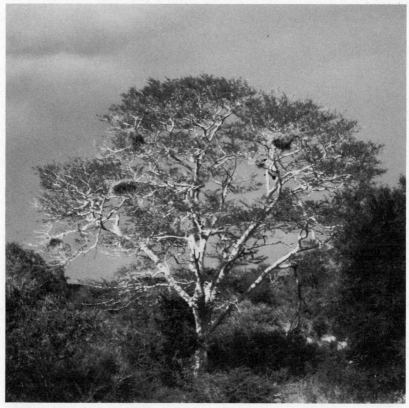

Acacia xanthophloea, the 'fever' tree as in 'The great grey-green, greasy Limpopo River, all set about with fever trees.' ('The Elephant's Child' – Rudyard Kipling.) The early explorers of Africa often slept by water under the fever tree and they frequently contracted malaria. This some attributed to an invisible 'miasma' from the tree.

FEVER AND ANTIPYRESIS

The role of the nervous system

KEITH E. COOPER

Professor Emeritus of Medical Physiology
University of Calgary, Canada

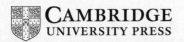

CAMBRIDGE
UNIVERSITY PRESS

Published by the Press Syndicate of the University of Cambridge
The Pitt Building, Trumpington Street, Cambridge CB2 1RP
40 West 20th Street, New York, NY 10011-4211, USA
10 Stamford Road, Oakleigh, Melbourne 3166, Australia

First published 1995

Printed in Great Britain at the University Press, Cambridge

A catalogue record for this book is available from the British Library

Library of Congress cataloguing in publication data

Cooper, K. E. (Keith Edward)
Fever and antipyresis : the role of the nervous system/ by Keith
E. Cooper.
    p.   cm.
Includes bibliographical references and index.
ISBN 0-521-41924-7 (hardback)
1. Fever – Pathophysiology.   2. Nervous system – Pathophysiology.
3. Body temperature – Regulation.   4. Pyrogens.   5. Antipyretics –
Mechanisms of action.   I. Title.
[DNLM: 1. Fever – physiopathology.   2. Fever – drug therapy.
3. Body Temperature Regulation – physiology.   4. Body Temperature
Regulation – drug effects.   5. Nervous System – physiopathology.
6. Pyrogens.   7. Anti-Inflammatory Agents, Non-Steroidal.   WB152
C777f 1995]
RB129.C66   1995
616' .047–dc20   94-42722 CIP
DNLM/DLC
for Library of Congress

ISBN   0 521 41924 7   hardback

To all of my colleagues with whom I have had the privilege of working on fever, and especially to Eileen for her support over the years.

Contents

Preface

In the past decade there have been excellent reviews of various aspects of the fever process. These include Moltz (1993), Kluger (1991a), Kluger (1991b), Hellon *et al.*, (1991), Blatteis (1990a,b), Coceani (1991), Stitt (1993) and an older one – Cooper (1987). Some have dealt with the immunological aspects, some with parts of the role of the central nervous system and some with the more general evolutionary aspects of the whole fever process. It was felt worth-while to discuss the role not only of the central nervous system but also of the peripheral nervous system in the development of the febrile response, and to add something of the problems which can arise in the nervous system as a result of fever. Our knowledge of the function of the nervous system in the genesis of fever has changed greatly in the last decade or so, and the extension of the participation of central nervous structures outside the hypothalamic area, in fever, has received attention.

Our understanding of the mechanisms of action of antipyretic drugs has been extended in the last few years, and a new concept of endogenous antipyresis has grown up in the last two decades. The role of the central nervous system in this is of paramount importance.

This book tries to present a synopsis of older and more recent information on the activity of the central and peripheral nervous systems in the many responses of the organism to infection and pyrogens. It is meant as a text for those interested in fever, its value and its draw-backs, whether they are graduate students, those engaged in academic medicine, advanced medical students, and perhaps to give a wider overview to those engaged in deeper studies of only one or two aspects of the fever process.

It was felt necessary to give some introductory outlines of the concepts of fever and the acute phase response, the relevant anatomical information and the processes of normal thermoregulation. There is, I hope, enough information in the introductory chapters, and Appendix 1, for those not directly involved in the field to be able to follow the later arguments. In the last chapter I have tried to summarize and co-ordinate the information available at the time of publication, and to add some deliberate speculations and suggestions for further studies.

The field which has changed out of all recognition in the last half century, after the epoch-making discovery of endogenous pyrogen by Paul Beeson, is still expanding rapidly. Naturally, I have given some space to the exciting work which my colleagues and I have enjoyed over the last few decades; but I hope that it has been kept sufficiently in the context of the other aspects of fever studied elsewhere. However, the present stocktaking will, I hope, provide a base for those who will advance the field further in the next generation. To paraphrase a Biblical comment (Joel, 2.28), I hope that while the old men dream dreams the young men will see visions and push our branch of science ahead. If this book helps them it will have been worth while. Much of what is discussed is still controversial and some of the readers on reading it may feel, as did Job in another context, 'my desire is that the Almighty would answer me and that mine adversary had written a book' (Job, 31.35, King James version). The hypotheses of today are but temporary structures to be replaced or modified if scientific knowledge is to advance, and to those younger workers who will do this I extend my best wishes.

Keith E. Cooper

Acknowledgements

The author wishes to thank his colleagues Drs. Veale, Pittman, Kasting, Naylor, Wilkinson, Poulin and many others for their permission to discuss their work in detail; Dr. Pittman for critical comments on the manuscript of this book; to Mrs Donna Shaw and Mrs Grace Olmstead for their great help with the preparation of the manuscript; to Mrs Rita Owen whose copy-editing greatly improved the manuscript; and to Jody Wood for compiling the index. The following publishers are acknowledged with many thanks for permission to reproduce figures in this book:
Academic Press, Fig. 2.4; Athlone Press, Fig. 2.5; Blackwell Scientific Publications, Figs. A1.4, A1.5, A1.6; Wm. C. Brown, Fig. 7.4; Churchill Livingstone, Figs. 2.8, 3.1; Marcel Dekker, Fig. 5.7; Mallincrodt Inc, Fig. 7.7; Oxford University Press, Fig. 4.2; Pergamon Press, Verbatim extract from Himms-Hagen; Raven Press, Fig. 5.5; W. B. Saunders, Fig. A1.7; Springer-Verlag, Table 6.2, Fig. 2.3; and the publishers of the following journals: *Acta Paedr. Scand.*, Fig. 8.1; *Amer. J. Physiol.*, Figs. 5.9, 7.8, 7.10; *Brain Res.* Tables 5.1, 5.2. Figs. 7.6, 8.2; *Brain Res. Bull.*, Fig. 7.4; *Clinical Science*, Figs. 1.1, 1.2, 1.3, 1.4, 1.5, 3.2; *Federation Proceedings*, Table 5.3; *J. Physiol. (Lond)*, Figs. 2.2, 4.1, 6.1, 6.2, 7.3, 7.5; *Lancet*, Table 6.1; *Peptides*, Fig. 7.9; *Physiol. Rev.*, Fig. 5.8; *Science*, Figs. 1.6, 1.7; *Yale J. Biol. Med.*, Figs. 5.4, 5.6, Table 1.1., and the authors from whose works the figures or tables are quoted and who are named either in the figure or table legend or are quoted in the appropriate text.

Glossary of acronyms

α-MSH	α-melanocyte stimulating hormone
AV3V	anteroventricular region of the third cerebral ventricle
aCSF	artificial cerebrospinal fluid
ACTH	adrenocorticotrophic hormone
AH/POA	anterior hypothalamus/preoptic area
AMP	adenosine monophosphate
AVP	arginine vasopressin
BAT	brown adipose tissue
BST	bed nucleus of the stria terminalis
CNS	central nervous system
CRF	corticotrophin releasing factor
CSD	cortical spreading depression
csf	cerebrospinal fluid
HRP	horseradish peroxidase
5-HT	5-hydroxytryptamine (serotonin)
ICP	intracranial pressure
icv	intracerebroventricular/ly
IFN	interferon
IL-1	interleukin-1
IL-6	interleukin-6
ip	intraperitoneal/ly
iv	intravenous/ly
kDa	kilo-Dalton
LAF	lymphocyte activating factor
LCVP	lateral cerebral ventricular pressure
LEM	leucocyte endogenous mediator
MEA	medial amygdaloid nucleus
MIP	macrophage inflammatory protein
MSG	monosodium glutamate

NTS	nucleus of the tractus solitarius
OVLT	organum vasculosum of the lamina terminalis
P_aCO_2	partial pressure of carbon dioxide (arterial blood)
PCPA	parachlorophenylalanine
PGD	prostaglandin D
PGE	prostaglandin of the E series
PGE_1	prostaglandin E_1
PGE_2	prostaglandin E_2
PGF	prostaglandin F
Poly I : Poly C	polyinosinic-polycytidylic acid
PVN	paraventricular nucleus
RES	reticuloendothelial system
SAE	*Salmonella abortus equi*
TNF	tumour necrosis factor
vcsf	ventricular cerebrospinal fluid
VSA	ventral septal area

1

Fever – definition, usefulness, ubiquity

What is fever?

While fever has been recognized as an important symptom of disease for millennia, the role of the nervous system in its induction has only really been investigated seriously in the present century. But, before examining this role it is necessary to define fever and to discuss matters such as its survival value and how widespread its occurrence is in the animal kingdom.

Two terms are commonly used to refer to a rise in the temperature of the body core namely, hyperthermia and fever. For the purposes of this book I will refer to fever as a rise in core temperature occasioned by a pathological process, in which the raised core temperature is defended. This condition could include the fevers related to that usually ill-defined condition 'stress'. Hyperthermia includes the condition of raised body temperature in the absence of a pathological process such as can be caused by immersion in a hot pool, or working in a vapour impermeable suit in the heat. The concept of a defended raised temperature, or raised set point, was clearly stated by Liebermeister, (1871). He wrote (in old German spelling): *'Der wesentliche Unterscheid des Fieberkranken vom Gesunden besteht demnach weder in der höheren Körpertemperatur noch in der grösseren Wärmeproduction, sondern darin, dass Wärmeverlust und Wärmeproduction für einen höheren Temperaturgrad regulirt werden. Zum Wesen des Fiebersgehört, dass die Wärmeregulirung auf einen höheren Temperaturgrad eingestellt ist'.*[1]

---

[1] 'The significant difference between the feverish person and the healthy one lies, therefore, neither in the higher temperature nor in the increased heat production, but in the fact that heat loss and heat production are regulated for a higher temperature level. It is part of the character of fever that heat regulation is set for a higher temperature level.'

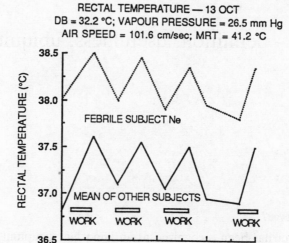

Fig. 1.1. Experiment illustrating that a febrile subject regulates body temperature during fever, albeit the level of temperature regulation is set higher both
at rest and during exercise. DB = dry bulb temperature; MRT = mean radiant
temperature. (From MacPherson, 1959, redrawn by Stitt, 1993.)

Jules Lefèvre (1911) wrote '*La fièvre est donc bien un trouble de la
régulation*', and referred to a person in a fever as having 'a new level
of temperature'. Richet (quoted in Lefèvre, 1911) immersed febrile
subjects in cool water which caused transitory reductions in body
temperature which returned to the same febrile level after the immersion. Later evidence for a raised body temperature set point in human
fever has come from Fox & MacPherson (1954), MacPherson (1959) and
Cooper *et al.* (1964c). Fox & MacPherson took the opportunity to study
a young man who was febrile as a result of a mild respiratory tract
infection. He was exercised periodically in a hot room over a period of
four hours, and his rectal temperature and sweat rates were monitored.
The same variables were measured under the same conditions when he
was afebrile. The changes in rectal temperature are shown in Fig. 1.1.
The exercise induced rises in core temperature in the febrile condition
which were closely similar to those seen in the afebrile subjects and the
sweating responses were also almost identical. The results are consistent
with the notion that his body temperature set point was raised during
the fever, and the work illustrates the need to be able to make

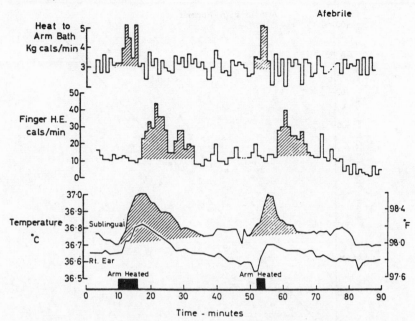

Fig. 1.2. Response of a normal subject to immersion of an arm in a warm water bath. Upper line indicates the electrical consumption of the bath (expressed as kg cals/min), shaded areas indicating the increment measuring the amount of heat taken up by the subject. The responses of finger heat elimination (H.E.) and sublingual temperature are indicated by shaded areas. (From Cooper *et al.*, 1964c.)

opportunistic observations provided by natural disturbances. Cooper *et al.* (1964c), studied the peripheral circulatory response to raising the body temperature by immersing one arm in warm water. The raised body temperature stimulated central warm receptors in such a way that the finger blood flow, as estimated by finger heat elimination, in the fingers of the unheated hand rose (Fig. 1.2). The area beneath the rise and fall in sublingual or auditory meatus temperature could be used as a measure of the stimulation of the central warm receptors, and the area beneath the rise and fall in finger heat elimination over the same period was an index of the effector response to that stimulation. Using varying periods of body heating it was possible to construct a graph of the relationship between the central warm receptor stimulation and the peripheral blood flow response. The relationship was significant and linear (Fig. 1.3). Eight subjects with febrile diseases had 27 arm immersions and their responses measured during fever (Figs. 1.4 and

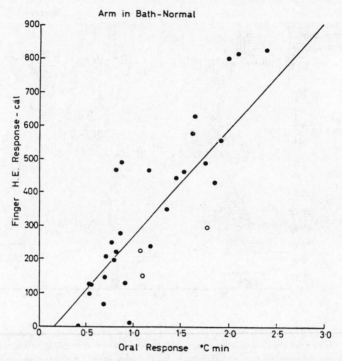

Fig. 1.3. The relation between oral temperature responses and finger heat elimination responses in afebrile subjects. Open circles represent results from one subject whose ear temperature was used instead of oral temperature. The regression line is shown. (From Cooper *et al.*, 1964c.)

1.5). The relationship between the central warm receptor stimulation and the blood flow response was virtually identical to that in the afebrile state. This provided further evidence to suggest that the warm receptor/peripheral vasodilatation mechanism functions normally in fever, but at a new set level.

The acute phase response

While much work has until recently concentrated only on the rise in body temperature in fever, it has been realized, more and more, that the temperature response is but one part of a complex host defence response to infection. This reaction is termed the *acute phase response*. In addition to the rise in body temperature the acute phase response includes an

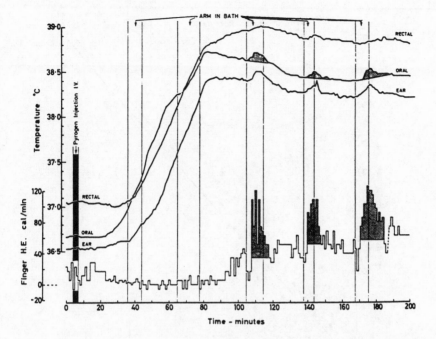

Fig. 1.4. Responses of temperature and heat elimination in a normal subject injected with pyrogen. Responses of oral temperature and heat elimination (H.E.), during stable temperature periods, are shaded. (From Cooper *et al.*, 1964c.)

initial fall in the neutrophil count which reaches a minimum in about one hour and is followed by a neutrophilia which is at a maximum at six hours and lasts for up to 24 hours (Cannon *et al.*, 1992). There is also a fall in the lymphocyte and monocyte counts and the fall in T cells is most marked (Richardson *et al.*, 1989). There is a fall in plasma iron (Elin & Wolff, 1974) which may be in part due to release of lactoferrin, an iron binder, during neutrophil degranulation (Weinberg, 1984). The fall in plasma iron may help to reduce bacterial replication by depriving them of an essential nutrient. There is also a reduction in the plasma zinc level which is not dependent on body temperature (Kampschmidt & Upchurch, 1970; Hacker *et al.*, 1981; Van Miert *et al.*, 1984). The reductions in plasma iron and zinc levels were found (Van Miert *et al.*, 1984) to occur in goats in response to tick-borne fever, staphylococcal enterotoxin and *Escherichia coli* endotoxin. There was evidence of a fall in plasma iron but either a rise or no change in plasma zinc in response

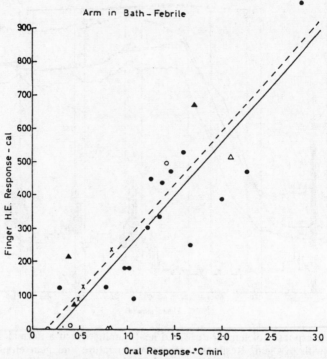

Fig. 1.5. The relation between oral temperature responses and finger heat elimination (H.E.) responses in subjects with febrile illnesses and febrile healthy subjects (solid circles). The solid line is the regression line for these points; the interrupted line is the regression obtained on afebrile subjects. Open circles and crosses represent observations on patient J.P. on two days. Solid triangles represent observation on patient M.H. during a stable fever, and open triangles observations while her temperature was rising. (From Cooper et al., 1964c.)

to trypanosomiasis and no significant changes in response to goat endogenous pyrogen. It is suggested that the plasma zinc and iron levels are regulated by different mechanisms and that different cytokines may, during fever, regulate the two trace metal levels in the plasma. The function of changes in plasma zinc levels in the acute phase response is not clear.

The effect of the rise of body temperature on host defence responses is complex. The basal metabolism of the organism changes with temperature with a Q_{10} of 2.1–2.3 in the human (Hockaday et al., 1962). A rise in core temperature would increase leucocyte mobility, possibly increase bactericidal activity and enhance lymphocyte transformation, with more controversial effects on such functions as antibody production

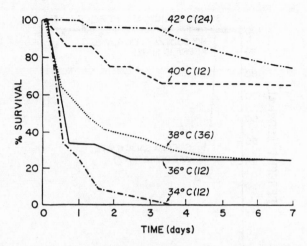

Fig. 1.6. Percentage survival of desert iguanas (*Dipsosaurus dorsalis*) infected with *Aeromonas hydrophila* and maintained at temperatures of 34 ° to 42 °C. The number of lizards in each group is given in parenthesis. (From Kluger *et al.*, 1975.)

and phagocytic activity of leucocytes (Kluger, 1981). There is in fever a rise in plasma copper, fibrinogen, RNA synthesis in the liver and plasma acute-phase globulins (see Kluger, 1981).

Endotoxin administration in the human induces many responses from the endocrine systems. These include a rise in plasma adrenaline in the early phase of fever, a rise in plasma noradrenaline, increases in plasma ACTH and cortisol and an increase in plasma growth hormone levels (see Cannon *et al.*, 1992).

Survival value of fever

There is a large body of evidence that behavioural fever in ec-totherms and fever in endothermic mammals assists survival in the face of infection. This was fully discussed first by Kluger (1979) in his monograph on fever. The effect of maintaining desert iguanas (*Dip-sosaurus dorsalis*) infected with *Aeromonas hydrophila* (an organism pathogenic to the species) at various environmental temperatures, on survival is shown in Fig. 1.6, which is taken from the classic paper of Kluger *et al.* (1975). Normally these creatures use behavioural shuttling between sun and shade to raise their temperatures in response to infection. In the experiment shown in Fig. 1.6 the animals were

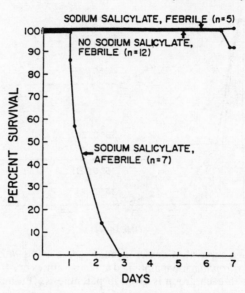

Fig. 1.7. Percentage survival rate of desert iguanas (*Dipsosaurus dorsalis*) infected with *Aeromonas hydrophila* with and without administration of sodium salicylate. (From Bernheim & Kluger, 1976b.)

artificially maintained at the various temperatures shown and it can be seen that the higher the lizard's temperature the greater the chance of survival. At 42 °C the survival rate at three to four days post-infection was near 90% and at body temperatures of 34 °C the mortality was 100%. Administration of the antipyretic, sodium salicylate, to desert iguanas infected with *A. hydrophila* severely reduces survival (Bernheim & Kluger, 1976b; see Fig. 1.7). The mortality was not due to salicylate toxicity. Other ectotherms have been demonstrated to have higher survival rates if behavioural fever is permitted to occur. The effect of fever on survival in the *Pasteurella multocida* infected rabbit was studied by Kluger & Vaughn (1978). Again it was shown that there was a good correlation between fever magnitude and survival up to body temperature increases of 2.25 °C, above this the survival rate declined. They also found that a mixture of sodium salicylate and acetaminophen, while preventing the very high fever due to large doses of bacteria, increased overall survival. Nevertheless this led to more animals being in the lower range of fever and to more animals in this range dying, but the percentage survival was greater than in controls in the same range. This suggested an effect of the drugs outside the temperature raising mechanism, possibly on the animal's immune responses. Salicylate given by microinfusion into the AH/POA (Vaughn *et al.*, 1980), in *P. multocida* infected rabbits, reduced the body temperature in the first five hours of infection. Rabbits, after having infusions of salicylate, had initially lower temperatures, but later increased fevers and higher mortalities than those infused with a control solution, and again there was a peak fever above which mortality increased. In a similar study (Vaughn *et al.*, 1981) rabbits infused with salicylate had reduced white cell counts and higher numbers of bacteria in the lungs and livers. The ability of the RES to clear particulate material was unaffected by the salicylate as was the intracellular viability of the organisms. This study again emphasizes the possibility of an action of the fever mechanism within the brain which leads to enhanced host defence reactions.

The above observations not only indicate an important role for fever in enabling the animal to resist infection but also indicate the danger of excessive fever. In most instances there seems to be an upper limit to fever in infection such that the body temperature does not reach a level at which temperature effects *per se* are lethal. This consideration has been in the minds of those who have acquired evidence for and postulated the existence within the brain and peripherally of endogenous antipyretic systems to act as brakes on the fever height and duration. There is always the danger in teleological thinking of assuming that all apparently useful adaptations have evolved by design, and then extending the evidence to cover all species and conditions. The ubiquity of fever has been challenged and the arguments concerning this follow in the next section. The concept of endogenous antipyresis is discussed in Chapter 8.

The ubiquity of fever

Fever occurs in response to infection or challenge with endotoxins in most endotherms by a combination of physiological (or 'autonomic') and behavioural mechanisms, and in many ectotherms by behavioural means. Cabanac & LeGuelte (1980) showed that scorpions can develop behavioural fever in response to PGE_1, and Bronstein & Conner (1984) observed behavioural fever in the Madagascar cockroach (*Gromphadorhina portentosa*) in response to endotoxin. The crayfish (*Cambarus bartoni*) also can develop fever in response to PGE_1 (Casterlin & Reynolds, 1978). Moving to vertebrates, the classical work of Bernheim & Kluger (1976a) demonstrated that both the desert iguana and the

Table 1.1. *Febrile responses of ectothermic vertebrates and invertebrates*

Species	Activator of fever
Reptiles	
Dipsosaurus dorsalis	Bacteria, IL-1
Iguana iguana	Bacteria
Terrepene carolina	Bacteria
Chrysemys picta	Bacteria
Amphibians	
Hyla cinerea	Bacteria
Rana pipiens	Bacteria
Rana catesbeiana	Bacteria
Rana esculenta	Bacteria, PGE_1, IL-1?
Necturus maculosus	PGE_1
Fishes	
Micropterus salmoides	Bacteria
Lepomis macrochirus	Endotoxin, bacteria
Carassius auratus	Endotoxin, bacteria
Invertebrates (arthropods)	
Cambarus bartoni (crayfish)	Bacteria
Gromphadorhina portentosa (cockroach)	Endotoxin, bacteria
Homarus americanus (lobster)	PGE_1
Penaeus duorarum (shrimp)	PGE_1
Limulus polyphemus (horseshoe crab)	PGE_1
Buthus occitanus (scorpion)	PGE_1
Androctonus australis (scorpion)	PGE_1

green iguana (*Iguana iguana*) could mount a behavioural fever, when allowed to shuttle between unheated areas and those heated by heat lamps, after inoculation with dead pathogenic bacteria. They were also able to show that the leucocytes from desert iguanas produced a pyrogen resembling other known endogenous pyrogens (Bernheim & Kluger, 1977). There is also evidence that tadpoles and tree frogs can develop fever in response to injection of pathogenic bacteria (Kluger, 1977; Casterlin & Reynolds, 1977). There is evidence that frogs can produce an endogenous pyrogen (Myhre *et al.*, 1977). Fishes also can respond to infection with behavioural fevers (Reynolds *et al.*, 1976). The responses to injected bacteria, endotoxins and prostaglandins in fishes, amphibia, reptiles and arthropods are given in Table 1.1 (taken from Kluger, 1986). Based on information of this kind it has been proposed that the ability to develop fever, and possibly the ability to generate other aspects of the acute phase response, developed early in the course of evolution, and that it has been preserved as a survival adaptation.

Many ectotherms from Africa do not develop behavioural fevers. Laburn *et al.* (1981) were unable to induce fever in a cordylid lizard (*Cordylus cataphractus*) in response to pyrogens. Similarly, endotoxin, killed staphylococci or killed *Salmonella minnesota* did not induce fever in the leopard tortoise (*Geochelone pardalis*) (Zurovsky *et al.*, 1987c). Two African snakes, *Psammophis phillipsii* and *Lamprophis fuliginosus*, also failed to respond with fever to bacterial pyrogens or killed organisms, (Zurovsky *et al.*, 1987a). Marx *et al.* (1984) reported a fish in which neither endotoxin nor PGE_1 produced behavioural fever. A study of ectotherms from the Namib desert, important because they maintain daytime core temperatures which are higher than most other ectothermic species, found that one beetle, *Onymacris plana*, did tend to select a warmer thermal preferendum after large doses of endotoxin, but two lizard species (*C. cataphractus* and *Aposaura anchietae*) did not respond to potential pyrogens (Mitchell *et al.*, 1990).

Thus it is not possible to conclude a ubiquitous evolution of the fever response to pyrogenic stimulation, and much more has to be done to determine whether the other beneficial acute phase responses can develop in some of the species which do not get fever. The whole exciting problem of the selection of fever and other beneficial acute phase responses is open to study on a comparative basis on many more species than at present reported, and the temptation to extrapolate from a relatively few species to a general evolutionary thesis will have to be shunned for the present. One interesting suggestion made by Cabanac & Rossetti (1987) as a consequence of their observation that snails do not get fever, was that the ability to respond with fever might have arisen between the appearance of the gastropods and the emergence of scorpions, i.e., between the Early Cambrian and the Late Silurian – an interesting research field for evolutionary biologists. The ability of such animals as arthropods to seek out warmer places and to raise their temperatures should provoke research on the neuronal mechanisms which could be studied electrophysiologically in their less complex neural networks.

Another cause of a rise in body core temperature is known as 'stress hyperthermia'. It was well described by Renbourn (1960). Youths in boxing clubs had little if any stress hyperthermia before practice bouts, but when awaiting a bout at the national championships, experienced this type of rise in core temperature. Psychological 'stress' in rats results in a rapid rise in body temperature which can be blocked or attenuated by icv administration of salicylate or intraperitoneal indomethacin (Kluger *et al.*, 1987; Moltz, 1993). Since 'stress' hyperthermia can be greatly attenuated by these PGE synthesis inhibitors it is suggested that a component of this type of hyperthermia could be a true fever.

Moltz (1993) also makes the case that neurogenic fever, that is the fever following cerebral emboli, neurosurgery and brain injury, is a true fever with a defended core temperature and that it appears to be PGE mediated.

2
Thermoregulation – an outline

Core temperature in various species

The range of body core temperature is, in most mammals, closely regulated. This is also true of birds. In many ectotherms, species which were once classified as poikilotherms, a relatively stable body core temperature is achieved during the daytime by shuttling between warmer and cooler regions, i.e., by a behavioural means. The regulated core temperatures vary with the species, and some of these ranges are shown in Table 2.1. In this Chapter I propose to give a sufficient outline of current thinking on the mechanisms of normal thermoregulation to enable the non-specialist reader to follow the later chapters on the disordered thermoregulation of body temperature which occurs in fever. It is not intended to give a full account of the details of all parts of the thermoregulatory neural mechanisms, or to detail the arguments for and against such things as the concept of 'set point'. These matters would require a book in themselves, and the reader is referred to such texts as Bligh (1973), Boulant et al. (1989), Schönbaum & Lomax (1990), and Gisolfi et al. (1993).

Sites of temperature measurement

There are several sites at which body temperatures are measured, especially in mammals. There is probably not a single temperature site which gives a measurement common to all of the body core. The rectal temperature is warmer than the oesophageal and mouth temperatures by about 1 °C. This does not appear to be related to bacterial action in the rectum (Cranston, personal communication) since the rectal temperature in a patient with a colostomy, and in whom the lower part of

Table 2.1. *The core temperature ranges for various vertebrates and invertebrates*

Animals	Core temperature (°C) range or preferred	Information source
Ectotherms (daytime):		
Desert iguana	39 ± 1	Kluger, 1979
Bullfrog	28	Kluger, 1979
Snakes – *Psammophis phillipsii*	33	Zurovsky *et al.*, 1987b
– *Lamprophis fuliginosus*	25	Zurovsky *et al.*, 1987b
Mammals:		
– eutherian	38 ± 2	Schmidt-Nielsen, 1975
– marsupial	36 ± 2	Schmidt-Nielsen, 1975
Others, e.g.,		
Cape golden mole	24–38	Withers, 1978
Namib golden mole	21–38	Fielden *et al.*, 1990
Birds	40 ± 2	Schmidt-Nielsen, 1975
Monotremes	31 ± 2	Schmidt-Nielsen, 1975
Invertebrates:		
Grasshopper	34	Boorstein & Ewald, 1987
Paramecium	24–28	Mendelssohn, 1902

the colostomy had been sterilized with antibiotics, was still higher than that in the oesophagus or mouth. There is evidence that the rectal mucosa can produce heat (Grayson, 1951; Malkinson *et al.*, 1978). The oral temperature can be useful especially if the mouth has been kept closed and no drinks or food have been taken for an hour or more (Gerbrandy *et al.*, 1954b). Mouth and oesophageal temperatures follow rapid changes in 'body' temperature more accurately than does the rectal. The oesophageal temperature gives a good index of the heart temperature over a wide range (Cooper & Kenyon, 1957). The temperature in the auditory meatus, particularly close to the tympanic membrane, also follows rapidly induced 'body' temperature changes (Cooper *et al.*, 1964d). The tympanic membrane temperature is said to give a good index of the hypothalamic temperature (Benzinger & Taylor, 1963). This has been disputed, but Cabanac (personal communication) has produced evidence in favour of the concept, provided that the measurement is made only on one small segment of the membrane. For practical purposes, when following the relatively slow core temperature changes in fever, any of the above loci of measurement can be used, provided that the same locus is used for the period of observation, to follow the trend in core temperature even though there will be absolute differences between different parts of the body core.

Core temperature and 'set point' concept

The regulation of the 'core' temperature in mammals with a narrow range of temperature regulation is the result of a complex interaction between thermal sensors, efferent heat retaining and dissipation and heat production mechanisms, and a central controller as yet not clearly identified. Under healthy conditions displacement of core temperature by artificial heating, cooling or exercise is followed by activation of efferent systems which return the core temperature to close to its resting value, and this is held by many to imply that there is a temperature 'set point', or temperature level, which is closely defended with a special brain mechanism in place to do so. In view of the diurnal swing in core temperature, which may be as much as 1.5 °C, 'set point' mechanism must be subject to other brain influences, and in view of the change in core temperature at ovulation probably to hormonal changes. As can be seen from Table 2.1. mammals usually have resting daytime (or, in the case of nocturnal mammals, night-time) core temperatures ranging from 36–38 °C. An example of the diurnal swing in temperature of laboratory rats is shown in Fig. 2.1. Some mammals let their core temperatures fluctuate more widely, as for example Grant's golden moles (*Erimitalpa grantii*) in the Namib desert. If these insectivorous mammals are submerged in sand, the temperature of which is manipulated over the 23–33 °C range, their core temperature follows that of the sand temperature. In sand at constant temperature the mole can control its temperature fluctuations to occur over a similar range. This allows periods of torpor for energy saving and by using heat from the sand the animal requires little metabolic energy to warm up (Fielden *et al.*, 1990). They seem to lie between endothermy and ectothermy. Some mammals, such as camels, link the daily swing of core temperatures to the degree of body hydration in order to conserve water. Importantly, as we will see later, many ectotherms which do not possess the means of physiological thermoregulation using metabolic means to maintain constant core temperatures use behavioural mechanisms to keep a relatively constant core temperature at above the ambient temperature in the daytime. This

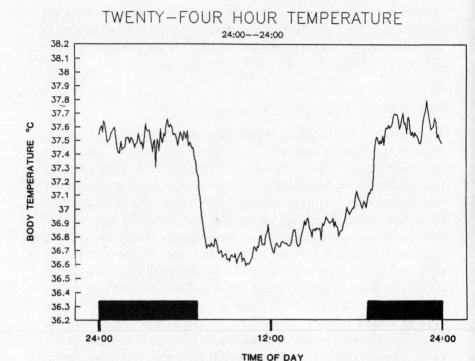

Fig. 2.1. The mean body temperature recordings of 16 adult Sprague Dawley rats measured over a 24-hour period. The ambient temperature was constant at 22 °C and the light controlled as shown. Dark bars indicate lights off (on 07.00, off 19.00). The activity pattern is closely similar. (T. J. Malkinson, Unpublished data.)

is achieved by such means as shuttling between the sun and the shade, or seeking a particular micro-environment or thermal preferendum. I will for the purposes of this book use the term 'fever' to mean a raised core temperature, apparently defended, caused by infection or other pathological process as opposed to the rise in temperature consequent upon exercise or body heating or cooling without pathological processes. There may be some overlap between the latter, which will be called 'hyperthermia', and fever by the above definition if pyrogenic cytokines are shown to be released, or endotoxaemia occurs in severe exercise. Fever, as defined in terms of a change in core temperature, is but one aspect of a more general defence response to infection and other disease processes which we now call the *acute phase response*, and which was described in greater detail in Chapter 1.

An outline of the mechanisms of temperature regulation

The control of body temperature requires at least three elements.

1. Means of detecting the core, surface and other internal temperatures.
2. Efferent systems to modify the heat production and the heat exchange with the environment.
3. Means of initiating and effecting responses to displacements in these temperatures.

Detection of surface and internal temperatures

There are many neuronal elements which have high thermosensitivities, i.e., greater than would be predicted by the simple effect of temperature on the cellular and membrane biochemical processes, and which are in some cases directional.

Thermoreceptors in the skin

There are two types of thermoreceptors in the skin, namely warm and cold receptors. Hensel (1981) lists the following characteristics specific to skin thermoreceptors: 'a. They have a static discharge at constant temperature (T); b. they show a dynamic response to temperature changes (dT/dt), with either a positive temperature coefficient (warm receptors) or a negative coefficient (cold receptors); c. they are not excited by mechanical stimuli; d. their activity occurs in the non-painful or innocuous temperature range'. The shape of the temperature/firing frequency plot for these receptors at steady temperatures is roughly bell shaped (Fig. 2.2, from Iggo, 1969). In the case of the warm receptors the firing rate increases as the temperature rises up to a peak value after which it decreases, and in the case of the cold receptors the firing rate increases as the temperature falls until a peak rate is reached after which the firing rate falls. A sudden change in temperature of the receptor induces a rapid (dynamic) firing response which settles down rapidly to the steady 'static' level determined by the new steady temperature (Fig. 2.3). Thus there are mechanisms to provide information not only about the level of skin temperature, but to detect sudden changes in surface temperature. The bell-shaped relationship between temperature and firing rate may be important in explaining some instances of paradoxical temperature sensations. There are many thermoreceptors in the skin with both types of receptors covering a fairly wide range of tempera-

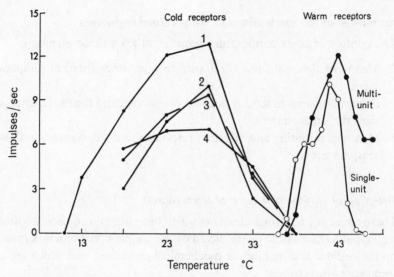

Fig. 2.2. Static firing rates of warm and cold responding cutaneous thermoreceptors plotted against receptor temperature. (From Iggo, 1969.)

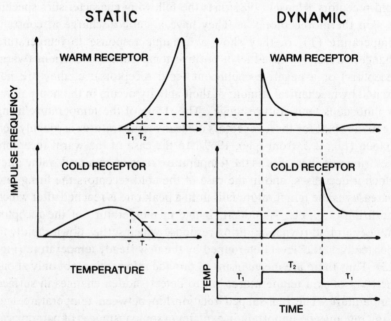

Fig. 2.3. On the left the receptor firing rates are plotted against the steady receptor temperature. On the right the firing rate of the receptors in response to abrupt changes of temperature are shown. (From Hensel, 1973b.)

tures. It has been suggested that the cold receptors lie deeper in the skin surface than do the warm receptors (Bazett & McGlone, 1930), but both are close to the surface. There is a higher density of cold than of warm receptors in the skin, and the density of both varies over the body surface. The weighting of skin areas used to calculate heat exchanges cannot be used to assess the contribution of thermal sensory inputs since the exact distribution of the superficial thermoreceptors over the whole of the body surface is not known precisely and may not follow the simple area pattern of heat exchange. The skin cold receptors are very dependent for their normal function on an adequate oxygenated arterial blood supply (Iggo & Paintal, 1977), and this together with the local temperature being outside the range of the cold receptor function may explain the failure of cold sensation in some cases of severe cold exposure. It is possible that the neural discharge patterns derived from the skin thermal receptors may not only supply the brain with information about the surface conditions of the body but also, if situated at various depths in the skin, about the surface heat fluxes. The skin temperature being highly dependent on the skin blood flow can also provide feedback information needed in the control of the skin circulation. For detailed analysis of the anatomy and neurophysiology of skin thermoreceptors the reader is referred to a monograph *Thermoreception and Temperature Regulation* (Hensel, 1981).

Thermoreceptors in the brain and spinal cord

There are highly thermosensitive neurons widely dispersed within the brain and spinal cord. The AH/POA has found a traditional place as a vital centre in thermoregulation. Most of the neurons in this region are not temperature sensitive, but there are both warm and cold sensitive neurons there (Nakayama *et al.*, 1963; Hellon, 1967). It has the highest density of thermosensitive neurons within the brain. It cannot be assumed that all highly thermosensitive neurons subserve thermoregulatory functions. Indeed, thermosensitivity may be a property common to many neural elements with some of them incorporated during evolution into the various hierarchies of temperature regulation.

The hypothalamic thermal detectors

Not only is the highest density of thermosensitive units in the central nervous system found in the hypothalamus but this region evokes the greatest systemic thermoregulatory response to local temperature change. Evidence for thermosensitivity in structures along the distribution of the internal carotid artery, in the rabbit, was obtained by Downey *et al.* (1964). By encircling various arteries with hollow clips which could be perfused with water at different temperatures they were able to alter the temperature of the blood coursing through the vessels. The greatest metabolic stimulation was obtained when the blood temperature in the internal carotid artery was lowered. Thermodes or diathermy devices positioned within the AH/POA have enabled those regions to be heated or cooled selectively (Magoun *et al.*, 1938; Hammel *et al.*, 1960; Andersson & Larsson, 1961; Ingram *et al.*, 1963). Many other references to hypothalamic heating and cooling are discussed by Bligh (1973).

In 1961 Nakayama *et al.* found that about 20% of hypothalamic neurons recorded in the anaesthetized cat were warm sensitive. Further analysis (Eisenman, 1972; Hellon, 1972) found three types of hypothalamic neuron randomly distributed which were thermally insensitive (60%), warm sensitive (30%) and cold sensitive (10%). Whether the responses to hypothalamic cooling result from decreased firing of warm sensitive neurons or to stimulation of cold firing neurones remains somewhat controversial (Hensel, 1981). There are also neurons, probably interneurons, that respond to altering the temperature at another locus, and some which respond to thermal stimulation of the body surface, e.g., scrotal skin. Others respond to heating and cooling of the spinal cord.

Combining the high thermal responsiveness of the AH/POA with the high density of thermosensitive neurons in that region it is reasonable to postulate that the thermosensitive units play a major role in body temperature regulation. Another mechanism of action of temperature changes could be high sensitivity of local neurotransmitter release to local temperature fluctuations, but such an explanation stretches the imagination. However, virtually nothing is known of the cytoarchitecture of the central thermoregulatory functions, and there is little evidence relating firing rates of AH/POA thermosensitive neurons to thermoregulatory behaviour in the awake, unrestrained, normally behaving animal, apart from the studies of Mercer *et al.* (1978) in the goat, and Hellon (1967), Reaves & Heath (1975) and Reaves (1977). These workers studied responses to hypothalamic temperature alterations in conscious animals, as opposed to the responses to naturally occurring changes in hypothalamic temperature in unrestrained animals exposed to various environmental conditions. Much more evidence is needed to confirm fully what at present seems the most reasonable hypothesis.

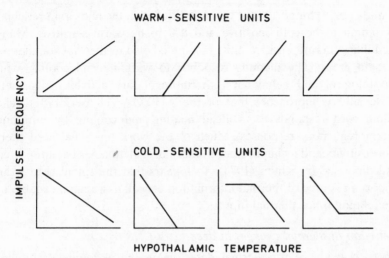

Fig. 2.4. Frequency/temperature curves for thermoreceptors found in the hypothalamus. (From H. H. Hensel, 1981.)

The hypothalamic thermosensitive neurons show a variety of firing patterns to local thermal stimulation. Some have linear temperature/firing rate relationships over a wide range of temperature, in some the slope is exponential and for others the relationship is non-linear or even discontinuous (Fig. 2.4). There are far fewer thermally sensitive neurons in the posterior hypothalamus, but there are some, and local heating there rather than initiating thermal responses can inhibit some previously generated thermal behaviours. There is also thermal sensitivity in the medial hypothalamus possibly related to behavioural thermoregulation.

The cerebral cortex
Thermoresponsive neurons were found in the cat sensorimotor cortex (Barker & Carpenter, 1970). As yet there is no evidence that they play a role in body temperature control. It is of interest that there is recent evidence that the frontal neo-cortex can exert a modulating effect on thermogenic activity evoked by lateral hypothalamic lesions (De Luca *et al.*, 1987), and can cause thermogenic activity when stimulated electrically (De Luca *et al.*, 1989).

The brain stem and spinal cord
There are both warm and cold sensitive neural units in the mid-brain reticular formation and in the medullary reticular formation. Hori &

Harada (1976) found 18% of the units studied in the mid-brain reticular formation to be cold sensitive and 8% to be warm sensitive. Many medullary thermosensitive units responded also to thermal stimulation of skin areas. The medulla responds to warming and cooling with physiological and behavioural thermoregulatory activities. Its thermosensitivity approaches that of the AH/POA (Hensel, 1981). The spinal cord responds to artificial heating and cooling by initiating thermoregulatory responses. Much of the work on spinal cord thermosensitivity and its importance in thermoregulation has been reported and discussed by Simon (1974). It appears that the spinal cord is an important source of thermal information as well as a region capable of modulating other thermal inputs.

Detection of thermal changes in deep extra-CNS regions

There is evidence for thermal detectors in the abdominal cavity of ruminants (Rawson & Quick, 1976). They were able to cause panting by intra-abdominal heating and to show that it was truly a response to heating structures within the abdominal cavity. It was suggested that the receptors lay in the walls of the intestine and rumen and possibly in the mesenteric veins. The thermal response to abdominal cooling does not appear to happen in rabbits or to heating and cooling in pigs (Ingram & Legge, 1972; Riedel et al., 1973). There may be some response to intragastric cooling in humans as a result of cooling of afferents from the stomach wall (Nadel et al., 1970). There is evidence for temperature sensitivity in some blood vessels and muscles (see Hensel, 1981), and that neurons subserving other functions can also show thermosensitivity, e.g., the carotid baroreceptors (Gallego et al., 1979).

Putative neurotransmitters

The presence of high concentrations of noradrenaline and 5-HT in the hypothalamus was demonstrated by Amin et al. (1954) and Vogt (1954). Using the formaldehyde condensation technique the presence of these amines in varicose terminals of neurons in the hypothalamus was established by Bertler (1961) and Carlsson et al. (1962). Both Brodie & Shore (1957) and von Euler (1961) suggested that the two amines could be involved in thermoregulation. On the basis of body temperature changes occasioned by injecting noradrenaline and 5-HT into the cerebral ventricles, or into the anterior hypothalamus of cats Feldberg & Myers (1963, 1965) proposed a new theory of temperature regulation.

It was that the core temperature depended on the balance between the two amines secreted into the hypothalamus. At a meeting of the British Physiological Society I asked Feldberg whether the theory was that there is release of monoaminergic neurotransmitters in synapses in the thermoregulatory circuits, or that he was postulating an interstitial amine 'soup' the content of which would modulate the activity of synaptic transmission. He opted for the neurotransmitter concept. Possibly a 'soup' notion would be considered more seriously now! In 1965, Cooper *et al.* published the results of injecting the same amines into the cerebral ventricles of rabbits. Whereas in the cat 5-HT raised and noradrenaline lowered body temperature, the opposite was found in the rabbit. Others followed, with some species responding to the monoamines in one way and others in the opposite (see Bligh, 1973). Bligh (1973) also proposed a neuronal model for sheep, goats and rabbits which used acetylcholine in synapses transmitting cold information and possibly heat production pathways and 5-HT in synapses transmitting warm information and possibly heat loss pathways with crossed inhibition possibly using noradrenaline. This model has been greatly expanded and is based on intraventricular or hypothalamic infusions of the amines. It has not yet been proved that the injected amines are acting on primary thermoregulatory circuits or whether they excite other non-thermoregulatory neurons which secondarily act on thermoregulatory neurons. In fact, we have little evidence with which to identify thermoregulatory neurons embedded in a mass of fibres subserving many functions in the hypothalamus.

There are several other possible neurotransmitter substances which could be used in thermoregulatory synapses, and these include dopamine and a variety of peptides. While some of these can, on local application within the brain, alter body temperature, the proof of their specificity as neurotransmitters in the thermoregulatory circuits needs further study.

Effector mechanisms in thermoregulation and their efferent systems

Two mechanisms are available to conserve or lose heat, namely behavioural and physiological. The former is of great importance in ectotherms and in many endotherms, and is a major component in human thermoregulation.

Behavioural thermoregulation

The principal means of temperature regulation which has enabled the human species to leave equatorial regions and colonize the more hostile northern and southern environments has been the ability to use and construct shelters and to make and use clothing. In this way control of the micro-environment has been regulated in the presence of severe conditions of temperature in the general environment. But, adopting particular patterns of behaviour is not confined to humankind. Many species of lizard can in the daytime shuttle between the shade and the sunlight, and by adjusting the time spent in each, can achieve a body core temperature well above the shady ambient temperature and so keep at maximum activity for catching prey. Other animals, e.g. fish, can seek out a preferred water temperature for maximum efficiency of their survival. Another behaviour is that of body orientation. An example of this is to be seen in the jack rabbit (*Lepus alleni*), sitting in the shade, with the position of its large ears set so that they radiate heat to the sunless part of the sky. Other animals may, in the heat, orientate their bodies so as to present minimal surface area to the solar radiation. A further mode is that of huddling together to share the heat of the whole group and insulating those in the middle of the huddle. In some newborn animals this behaviour not only contributes to keeping warm but reduces their energy expenditure (Mount, 1979). These are but few of the types of behavioural thermoregulation which, as we will see later, can be of great significance in fever. In endotherms there is co-ordination between behavioural and physiological thermoregulation with both usually being used at the same time.

Control of behavioural thermoregulation starts with detection of the environmental thermal conditions and the thermal topography of the body. Both hypothalamic and surface temperatures are used in causing behavioural thermoregulatory responses. By a combination of environmental temperature modification and hypothalamic heating Myhre & Hammel (1969) were able to show that both brain and peripheral temperatures were important in behavioural thermoregulation in the lizard, *Tiliqua scincoides*. Earlier, Cabanac *et al.* (1965) had shown that dogs changed (lowered) the preferred temperature of their environments by choosing the coolest of several enclosures when their core temperature was raised after drinking hot water. There are many reports of behavioural thermoregulatory corrective responses induced by altering the hypothalamic temperature (see Hensel, 1981, p. 186). Similarly, operant behavioural responses, e.g. bar pressing to select radiant heat bursts, have been demonstrated, in rats, in response to hypothalamic cooling (Satinoff, 1964). The confirmations of this result have been obtained in many species including primates.

Physiological or autonomic mechanisms

Heat production

Sources of heat production include the basal energy release resulting from the necessary cellular metabolism of the body tissues, the level of voluntary muscular activity, shivering thermogenesis and non-shivering thermogenesis. To these sources of heat must be added heat gained from solar radiation, from contact with warm objects such as electric blankets and heat gained by ingestion of warm food or drinks. The basal metabolic rate (cellular metabolism) is itself temperature dependent.

Basal metabolism

The Van't Hoff–Arrhenius relationship, which predicts the simple effect of temperature on cellular heat production as the result of heating or cooling on the biochemical reactions, applies to basal metabolism. This predicted change, which has been measured in poikilothermic animals, implies a change in O_2 consumption of between two and three times for every 10 °C change in body temperature. This change is termed the Q_{10} value. Measurements in one human in whom there were, as a result of hypothalamic disease, no active thermoregulatory responses gave a Q_{10} of 2.1–2.3 (Hockaday *et al.*, 1962).

The so-called basal metabolism, that is the energy release by metabolism at complete rest, both mentally and physically, in a neutral thermal environment and in a post-absorptive condition can be assessed by measuring the O_2 consumption. The condition is very difficult to achieve in practice, particularly in patients, and at one time the 'sedated' metabolic rate was used instead. This was measured in patients under maximal sedating doses of thiopentone, and gave more consistent data the meaning of which was sometimes questioned. However, the basal metabolism is mainly dependent on the circulating levels of the thyroid hormones, but can also be changed by drugs such as amphetamines or environmental pollutants such as cereal crop sprays containing dinitro-ortho-cresol (Bidstrup & Payne, 1951), which were used in Britain in the 1940s and 1950s. Some have standardized the conditions under which the resting metabolism can be measured as including being awake but fully relaxed and fasted for 12 hours in a thermoneutral environment, and this gives the minimum metabolic rate. Further modifications of the measurement of standard metabolic rate in infants have been described (Brück, 1978).

Active processes altering metabolism

Voluntary muscular activity

A well-used mechanism is raising or lowering the level of voluntary muscular activity. Relaxing, where possible in the heat, decreases metabolic rate, and muscular exercise in the cold produces increased heat. These responses really fall into the category of behavioural thermoregulation.

Shivering

The involuntary twitching of groups of muscles, which perform no useful work, in the cold is known as shivering. Shivering is a reflex response to lowering of both core and skin temperatures (Kleinebeckel & Klussman, 1990). Shivering can be induced by cooling the spinal cord and the hypothalamus (Simon, 1974). Heat production of the order of $300\,kcal.h^{-1}$ can be achieved by shivering in the human at ambient temperatures near $0\,°C$. The ability to shiver may take some days to develop after birth in the human baby (Brück, 1961), and is absent in many people over the age of 69 years (Collins *et al.*, 1977). Dogs with their spinal cords severed can, when the limbs are immersed in cold water, shiver in the muscles innervated from above the lesion (Sherrington, 1924). Observations in patients who had suffered complete spinal cord injuries found that they shivered during body cooling in the muscles innervated from above the level of cord severance even with the trunk skin temperature above $33\,°C$, and without feeling cold (Johnson & Spalding, 1974). These observations imply the existence of thermoreceptors within the central nervous system which can initiate shivering without cold receptor input from the periphery. The central nervous pathways involved in shivering are complex and include the septal region, the hypothalamus and the spinal cord. Andersson (1957) stimulated the septal region electrically in goats and found that this produced shivering, peripheral vasoconstriction and inhibited panting in heat exposed animals, and sometimes caused piloerection. The shivering and vasoconstriction were enough to induce a significant rise in the animals' core temperatures. Studies in which electrical stimulation of hypothalamic areas (Stuart *et al.*, 1961) and hypothalamic lesions were made (Stuart *et al.*, 1962) supported the view that the dorsomedial hypothalamus was a primary region in the initiation and maintenance of shivering, and that the septal region exerted a modulatory effect, with perhaps some ability to initiate shivering. It is also of interest that the baroreceptors and the chemoreceptors have been shown to influence shivering in the rabbit (Mott, 1963). Baroreceptor stimulation enhanced shivering and chemoreceptor stimulation suppressed it. It is therefore important in studies of the initiation and levels of shivering to ensure that such factors as blood pressure and blood chemistry do not confound the observations.

For a more detailed discussion of the neuronal mechanisms the reader is referred to Janský (1979) and Kleinebeckel & Klussman (1990).

The other major source of heat production during cold exposure in newborns and many adult animals, such as the rat and some hibernating species, is BAT. This specialized fatty tissue is found in the interscapular region, near the kidneys, in the thoracic cavity close to the heart and the aorta and sometimes in the inguinal region. It has an abundant vascularization with veins which drain the blood from it towards the central vital organs such as the heart. The fat globules are small and numerous. BAT has a rich sympathetic nervous innervation and has a high density of mitochondria. The sympathetic nervous innervation is β-noradrenergic. The nerve terminals contain neuropeptide Y in addition to noradrenaline. The following sequence of events between the activation of the sympathetic nerves to BAT and heat production is quoted verbatim from Himms-Hagen (1990):

a) Noradrenaline released from sympathetic nerves interacts with a β-adrenergic receptor;
b) adenylate cyclase activity increases and cyclic AMP level in the cell rises;
c) cyclic AMP stimulates the activity of a protein kinase that phosphorylates hormone-sensitive triacylglycerol lipase to produce the active form of this enzyme;
d) the rate of intracellular lipolysis increases and the fatty acid level rises;
e) the fatty acids have two functions, one to switch on the proton conduction mechanism by interacting with the uncoupling protein (UCP), the other to serve as the fuel for the increased thermogenesis;
f) dissipation of the proton gradient by increased operation of the proton conductance pathway increases the rate of operation of the electron transport system;
g) oxidation of fatty acids in the β-oxidation cycle and the tricarboxylic acid cycle

regenerates the reduced coenzymes oxidized in the electron transport system;

h) long-term stimulation leads to a cyclic AMP-mediated increase in synthesis of lipoprotein lipase, hence to increased extracellular lipolysis and substitution of fatty acids from blood lipids (very low density lipoproteins [VLDL] and chylomicrons) derived from the dietary carbohydrate and lipid for those derived from endogenous stores;

i) endogenous stores are also replenished by synthesis of fatty acids from glucose;

and

j) increased thermogenesis persists until the stimulus, noradrenaline, is removed, that is, until the increased sympathetic nervous system activity subsides.

BAT occurs in the newborn in many species, and in some, such as the rat, it persists as an important heat source into adult life. It is of great importance to hibernating animals as a source of heat during awakening from hibernation. The control of heat production by BAT involves the ventromedial hypothalamus, and there is some argument concerning the possible role of the dorsomedial hypothalamus and the paraventricular nucleus. Since many parts of the hypothalamus are involved in endocrine functions which play adjunct roles to thermoregulation one would expect that their interconnexions with the ventromedial hypothalamus would influence BAT metabolism. In fever the nucleus of the tractus solitarius is an important part of the sympathetic outflow which controls BAT activation. As with other aspects of thermoregulation the complexity of the hypothalamic and brainstem circuitry involved, and its close integration with other autonomic functions has made our understanding of the neuronal cytoarchitecture difficult to unravel, and for the most part we are grossly ignorant of the essential connectivities.

Heat elimination

The physical factors involved in heat loss or elimination are conduction, convection, radiation and evaporation. Heat conduction occurs between the body and any object with which it is in contact. Thus sitting on cold ground will drain heat from the body as will being immersed in cold water, and the heat flow will be proportional to the temperature difference between the body surface and the medium to which heat is lost. Convection involves the heating of the air, or other medium, at the body surface which becomes more buoyant, moves upward over the body surface and is replaced by cooler denser air. This process requires gravity and thus cannot take place in gravity-free conditions in space.

Wind blowing over a surface extracts heat by a process known as forced convection. Radiation is a major route of heat loss or gain. The exchange of heat is proportional to the differences in the fourth powers of the temperatures (in $°K = °C + 273$) of the radiating surface and the 'surface' with which radiation exchange takes place. Evaporation requires heat for the change in state, e.g. from water to water vapour and thus perspiration from the skin or respiratory tract is a very important means of losing heat. The heat loss amounts to 2421 kJ (or 576 kcal) for each 1 g of water evaporated at 30 °C. The full mathematical treatment of these physical routes of heat exchange are given in Kerslake (1972). The *heat balance equation* is:

Heat production ($M - W$) = $\pm R \pm C \pm Cd + E$ (heat loss) $\pm S$ (heat storage)

where M = metabolic heat production, W = external work, R = radiation heat exchange, C = convective heat exchange, Cd = conductive heat exchange, E = evaporative heat loss and S = heat storage. Cd is small except under special circumstances such as lying on the snow!

Heat loss from the skin is determined by the superficial skin temperature and this in turn is set by a combination of the environmental temperature and the *skin blood flow*. The neural control of the latter is of paramount importance and is mediated via the sympathetic nervous system. There are two main skin regions where the sympathetic nervous control differs. The skin of the hands and feet and to a lesser extent the distal parts of the forearms and the calves have a high density of arterio-venous anastomoses near the surface, and the vascular innervation is that of tonic vasoconstrictor impulses. Vasodilatation in these areas is achieved by release of vasoconstrictor tone, and the huge blood flows which can occur in the fingers, for example, happen by the opening up of the arterio-venous shunts. Though deeper in the skin than the surface capillaries, the extra tissue insulation above the shunts is more than compensated for by the much greater flow through the shunts as compared to that possible through the more superficial capillaries. An example of the levels of heat elimination at different distances from the finger tips in response to body heating is shown in Fig. 2.5 (Cooper, 1965a). Vasodilatation in the hand can be induced by raising the body temperature, for example by infusing warm saline intravenously (Gerbrandy *et al.*, 1954b) or immersing the opposite forearm and hand in warm water (see Fig. 1.2; Cooper *et al.*, 1964c). The warm stimulus to vasodilatation is linearly related to the vasodilator response over a

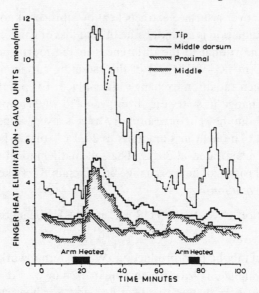

Fig. 2.5. Finger heat elimination from unit areas of the palmar surfaces of the proximal, middle and distal phalanges and the dorsum of the middle phalanx. The opposite arm was immersed in warm water at the times shown. (From Cooper, 1965a.)

wide range (Cooper *et al.*, 1964c). Pickering (1932) showed that putting one forearm and hand in warm water induced vasodilatation in the opposite hand, and that obstructing the circulation to the heated arm prevented this response, i.e., the response was not a reflex. Further evidence indicates that there are warmth receptors distributed along the course of the internal carotid artery in the human which mediate hand vasodilatation (Fig. 2.6). While there are no direct measurements of vasomotor responses to hypothalamic thermal stimulation in the human, there are numerous reports of this in other animals, and in addition to hypothalamic thermal stimulation, altering the spinal cord temperature can also induce vasomotor responses in animals. The analogy with other species would reasonably suggest the location of thermosensitive structures in the hypothalamus which could evoke responses in peripheral blood flow in the human. There is evidence (Cooper *et al.*, 1957) that the isolated human spinal cord does not contain thermosensitive structures which can evoke *efferent* nervous vasomotor responses.

A true reflex vasodilatation occurs in the hand if the front of the trunk is suddenly exposed to radiant heat (Fig. 2.7; Cooper & Kerslake, 1954). This reflex response involves afferent nerve fibres which appear to travel

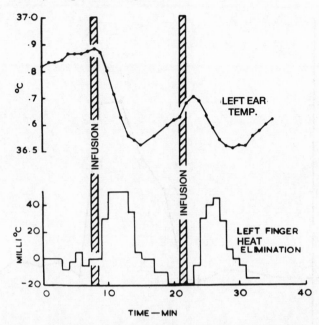

Fig. 2.6. Blood flow (heat elimination) in the fingers of the left hand, and left auditory meatus (core) temperature on infusion of warm saline into the right internal carotid artery in the human. Infusion time indicated by hatched columns. The induced vasodilatation led to a fall in core temperature as measured deep in the left auditory meatus. (Snell, Cranston & Cooper, unpublished observations.)

to the spinal cord in the sympathetic chain (Cooper & Kerslake, 1953), and possibly have a reflex arc which extends as far rostrally as the posterior hypothalamus (Rorstad, Korenblum & Cooper, unpub. data). The skin receptors do not appear to be those mediating conscious thermal sensation (Cooper & Kerslake, 1953; Appenzeller & Schnieden, 1963). The reflex vasodilatory response is quantitatively related to the radiant heat load. Reflex vasodilatation is usually inhibited at core temperatures below 36.5 °C and is progressively reduced at mean skin temperatures, in the heated area, below 33 °C (Cooper *et al.*, 1964b). The function of this reflex in modern clothed humans is difficult to assess. It could be a useful initial and short-term adjusting mechanism to sudden heat exposure. It is however a reflex useful in testing sympathetic function clinically, and in testing sympathetic efferent function in fever. The response is particularly marked in skin areas having many arterio-venous shunts.

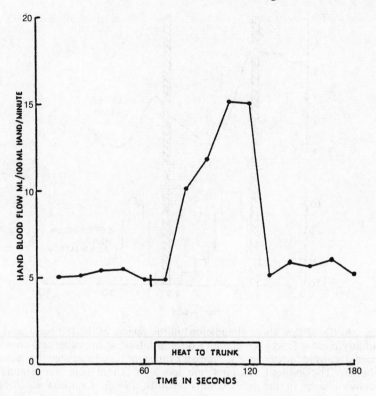

Fig. 2.7. Changes in hand blood flow on applying radiant heat to the trunk are shown. This curve is the mean of ten identical experiments. (From Cooper & Kerslake, 1954.)

The control of skin blood flow in the forearm and other more proximal areas involves active vasodilator nerves. These nerves are cholinergic. One mechanism has been postulated for active vasodilatation in the proximal and trunk skin regions, and this is the 'bradykinin' hypothesis. It suggests that cholinergic nerves to sweat glands evoke sweating and that the active sweat glands release into the tissue spaces enzymes which cause the formation of the vasodilator peptide bradykinin (Fox & Hilton, 1958). This would gear the blood flow to the metabolic needs of the active glands. This is an hypothesis which is poorly supported and against which there is much evidence. It appears that locally formed bradykinin could play a small role of regional skin vasodilatation but other mechanisms appear to be more important.

In addition to the effects of body core and reflex heating and cooling on the skin blood flow, local heating or cooling cause dilatation or constriction of the thermally stimulated skin. Severe cooling of the skin, particularly of the fingers, can lead to cold vasodilatation which occurs in waves (Lewis, 1930).

The second major component of heat loss from the skin is the evaporation of water from *sweat* on the skin and from that which diffuses through the skin – *insensible perspiration*. The lattter is determined by the difference in the water vapour pressures at the skin surface and the adjacent air, and is not under physiological control. The output of the sweat glands is under the control of cholinergic sympathetic nerves. The drive to sweating comes both from the warm receptors in the central nervous system and from warm receptors in the skin, the two inputs being integrated to determine the level of sweating. Stimulation of either can induce sweating depending on the level of the other (Hensel, 1981). In some species in which sweating either does not occur, or in which sweating is a minor route of heat loss, heat loss by *evaporation from the respiratory tract* is extremely important. Panting enables air to be moved rapidly over the upper respiratory evaporatory surfaces by very rapid shallow breathing, and this does not thus lead to respiratory alkalosis. It can be determined by peripheral heating since panting in sheep occurs during heat exposure without any change in temperature in the carotid artery; and if the central temperature is high enough also by anterior hypothalamic heating (Bligh, 1973).

Heat conservation

In the human there are three main mechanisms of heat conservation namely, behavioural, inhibition of sweating and skin vasoconstriction. The behavioural change includes adding more insulation over the body, raising the environmental temperature and postural change (such as assuming a foetal position) to reduce the surface area of skin exposed to the environment. Cessation of sweating requires the inhibition of the efferent sympathetic discharge to the sweat glands, and this occurs in response to skin cooling as well as to a fall in core temperature, or to a rise in the body temperature set point. It is interesting that sweating often occurs during sleep when the body temperature set point is lowered and ceases immediately on waking as the set point is abruptly raised. Vasoconstriction in the skin may be brought about by a local fall in the skin temperature over the same area, a fall in core temperature and with a rise in set point. There is a reflex skin vasoconstriction which is initiated by sudden cooling of quite a small area of skin, but this reflex

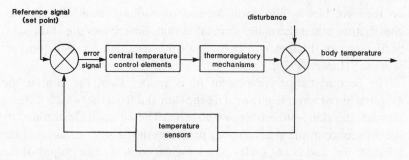

Fig. 2.8. Engineering model control system for thermoregulation.

reduction in skin blood flow is transient (François-Franck, 1876; Picker-ing, 1932). Reduction in core temperature is sensed by thermodetectors in the hypothalamus and also in the spinal cord, resulting in appropriate changes in sympathetic discharges to the skin blood vessels.

In other species the same modes of heat retention may be used together with piloerection – the raising of hair or fur to trap more air and increase body insulation – and a reduction in respiratory frequency with less air movement over the upper respiratory tract evaporatory surfaces.

The control systems in the central nervous system for thermoregulation

For the stable regulation of the temperature of a body of considerable mass and a varying heat production which is subject to large alterations in its thermal environment a precise feedback control system is required. Such a system, which is often postulated, is shown in Fig. 2.8. The regulator requires evidence of the set point to be defended, the state of the skin temperature and perhaps skin heat flux and the activity of the neurons controlling the heat loss and heat retention mechanisms. The difficulty is that the actual controller can only be described in terms of a 'black box' since the cytoarchitecture of the thermal control systems in the central nervous system is virtually unknown. The sources of thermal information from the body surface and the periphery have been described earlier in this chapter. We know that the hypothalamic region is crucial to thermoregulation since its destruction experimentally or by disease seriously impairs thermoregulation whereas lesions above the hypothalamus do not. We also know that neurons in the hypothalamus subserve many control functions such as water balance regulation, the control of endocrine functions, appetite control as well as thermoregulation, and the nerve fibres are intertwined rather than separated into discrete tracts as in the spinal cord. Thus, it is difficult to tease out and record the fibres involved in thermoregulation. Good observations on interconnections of thermosensitive neurons have been made in hypothalamic slice preparations, and some beginnings have been made in delineating the cytoarchitecture of these fibres (Boulant & Dean, 1987). It is but a beginning. Much has also been made of the thermoregulatory responses to the local hypothalamic application of monoamine neurotransmitters shown to occur in the varicose terminals of fibres in that region. The true explanation of such work awaits the more precise localization of the thermoregulatory neurons and methods for restricting the application of putative neurotransmitters to their synaptic regions. There is evidence for aminergic ascending pathways from the lower brainstem which are of importance in thermoregulation (Brück & Hinckel, 1980). It is also possible that the midbrain reticular arousal system could modify thermoregulatory behaviour. Bligh has also pointed out that there has to be crossed inhibition of heat loss and heat retention and heat production so that only the appropriate mechanism is functioning at any one time (Bligh, 1972). Myers & Veale (1971), using push–pull perfusion in the posterior hypothalamus obtained evidence for the ratio of potassium to calcium ions as a factor in determining the set point of body temperature. The interpretation is not universally accepted, but evidence for and against is still appearing in the literature. A further complication to the unravelling of thermoregulatory control systems are the inbuilt hierarchies of thermal control systems which have been preserved as the brain and spinal cord evolved (Satinoff, 1974). This means that some thermoregulatory function can be preserved by the action of lower regions of the brainstem in the presence of destruction more rostrally.

For the purposes of discussing the mechanisms of fever I will place the main region controlling thermoregulation in the AH/POA region with the efferent organization in the posterior hypothalamus, with further relays in the lower brainstem and spinal cord, and treat the set point mechanism and the controller as poorly understood black boxes.

3

The nature of pyrogens, their origins and mode of release

In the aphorisms of Sanctorious (Lister, 1701 in Sanctorii Sanctorii, 1701) we read '*In febribus intermittentibus cur perspiratio insensibilis prohibetur? quia humor peccans est in ambitu corporis*'. In other words 'Why is insensible perspiration (the term then for sweating) stopped in fever? because an evil humour circulates in the body'. This may be the earliest mention, in ignorance, of what we now call an endogenous pyrogen.

We now define a pyrogen as a substance which when introduced into the circulation, or given intracerebrally, causes the symptoms and consequences of fever, namely a rise in body temperature which at its plateau behaves as though the temperature is regulated, and which is brought about by a combination of heat retention processes and increased metabolic rate. The process which we have defined as fever is now thought to be but one part of a complex host defence reaction involving not only a rise in temperature but activation of many immune responses and processes for the destruction of micro-organisms. This process is termed the acute phase response. Pyrogens as defined above must be differentiated from substances which just affect the metabolic rate such as dinitro-ortho-cresol, or which cut down heat loss such as adrenergic agonists, but which do not induce the acute phase response. The rise in temperature caused by such agents should be termed hyperthermia, not fever, and the agents should be termed hyperthermic agents not pyrogens.

Pyrogens can be divided into those which are formed outside the body, the exogenous pyrogens, and those which are derived from body tissues within the body, the endogenous pyrogens. The endogenous pyrogens include fever producing cytokines which are peptides elaborated by cells such as monocytes and macrophages of the reticuloendothelial system.

Other endogenously produced substances such as prostaglandins play important roles in inducing fever.

Exogenous pyrogens

These may be derived from bacteria, fungi and other micro-organisms.

Bacterial pyrogens

The exogenous pyrogens which have received the most study in the last few decades are those derived from the cell walls of Gram-negative bacteria. They, by long usage of an inaccurate term, have come to be known as 'endotoxins'. These substances are large molecules having a molecular weight of about 1×10^6 daltons. They can be extracted from suspensions of Gram-negative bacteria by many methods (Work, 1971), but one method which enables a very pure product with little or no protein contamination to be obtained is by precipitation in a phenol/water mixture (Westphal & Luderitz, 1954). The endotoxin so extracted is a complex lipopolysaccharide made up of three moieties. Typically there is a basal core polysaccharide made up of sugars such as glucose, galactose, glucosamine, etc. and this is joined to a lipid component, the lipid-A, usually by a branched trisaccharide of 2-keto-3 deoxyoctonic acid (Fig. 3.1). The other moiety joined to the core polysaccharide is the O-specific side chain, made up of repeating units of oligosaccharides and which determines the antigenic properties of the endotoxin. It is the lipid-A part of the molecule which is principally responsible for the pyrogenic properties of the molecule (Luderitz *et al.*, 1973).

Repeated iv injection of the same dose of Gram-negative endotoxin, at daily intervals, results in progressively diminishing fever, particularly of the second phase of biphasic fever. This reduction in the extent of fever with the repeated injections is known as 'tolerance'. Tolerance is not a feature of repeated injection of 'endogenous pyrogen' (Bennet & Beeson, 1953a), or of the pyrogen extracted from fungi such as *Candida albicans* (Braude *et al.*, 1958).

While endotoxins may be altered, in part, by heat treatment, their pyrogenic action is remarkably heat stable, and when doing experiments on non-lipopolysaccharide pyrogens or injecting materials directly into the hypothalamus it is necessary to treat the glassware or cannulae by

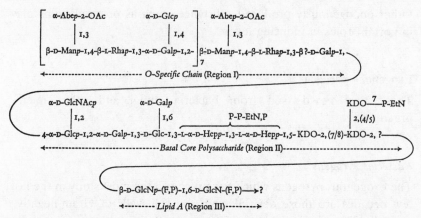

Fig. 3.1. Composition of a lipopolysaccharide from *Salmonella typhimurium*.
(From Work, 1971.)

heating to about 300 °C for several hours, or to boil them in alkali to
be absolutely certain that endotoxin contamination is avoided. Autoclav-
ing is not adequate for their destruction though it does attenuate the
fever response. Dry endotoxin can be stored for many months or even
years at temperatures of –15 °C or lower, and stock solutions can be kept
for a shorter time in the freezer.

Cell walls of some Gram-positive bacteria, e.g., streptococcus
pyrogens and some strains of staphylococci contain pyrogenic toxins the
chemical nature of which is not as fully explored as those from the
Gram-negative bacteria. They are capable of producing high biphasic
fevers and of inducing tolerance. The fever produced can be due either
to the direct pyrogenic action of the cell wall toxin, or to induced
antigen–antibody reactions. The cell wall pyrogens may act through a
different peripheral pathway, in inducing direct fever, from that used by
endotoxins. It is worthy of note that an organism which produces one
of the most severe fevers is the pneumococcus, a Gram-positive
bacterium.

It is also important to remember that killed bacteria can produce fever
when injected iv or into the hypothalamus, and in the early 1940s
repeated daily iv injections of typhoid vaccine were given to induce fever
and in order to reduce arterial blood pressure in cases of malignant
hypertension. It gave immunity to typhoid bacilli but had little lasting
effect on the blood pressure. The same treatment was also used for

cerebral syphilis in the days preceding the use of antibiotics, but the fever was more often induced by infecting the patient with the parasites of tertian malaria, or by whole body diathermy (Neymann, 1936)!

Fungal pyrogens

Braude *et al.* (1960) published an extensive study of the pyrogenic properties of four fungi. Living suspensions of *Candida albicans*, *Blastomyces dermatitidis*, *Histoplasma capsulatum* and *Sporotrichum schenckii* produced fever when injected iv into rabbits, but *Cryptococcus neoformans* did not. They noted two types of fever. The first was similar to that seen after Gram-negative endotoxin injection with a relatively rapid onset and depending on the dose monophasic or biphasic. The other started as long as 24 hours after the injection and was often followed by death. The pyrogen causing the first type of fever was heat stable, could be produced by cell-free filtrates of cultures, did not induce tolerance and did not cause shock in large doses. Immediate neutropaenia followed by neutrophilia followed injection. Apart from this series of experiments in which the release of endogenous tissue pyrogen was postulated to occur, the cytokine pathway of fungal pyrogen is still very much open to investigation.

A synthetic pyrogen

Abscher & Stineberg (1969) and Weinstein *et al.* (1970) showed that a synthetic double stranded helical RNA polymer namely, Poly I:Poly C is a potent pyrogen and induces tolerance. There is cross-tolerance to Gram-negative endotoxins. This substance may be of importance in the study of fever due to viral infections.

Endogenous pyrogens

A major turning-point in our understanding of the mechanism of fever, in this century, was the discovery by Beeson (1948) that granulocytes, obtained from peritoneal exudates which were not contaminated with bacterial pyrogen, could elaborate a pyrogen. In further studies, Bennet & Beeson (1953a,b) confirmed Beeson's initial observation and demonstrated that the pyrogen derived from leucocytes was heat labile, did not induce tolerance on repeated injection and would cause fever in animals made tolerant to bacterial pyrogen. In 1954, Gerbrandy *et al.*

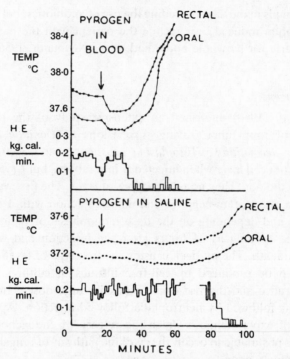

Fig. 3.2. The effect of bacterial pyrogen in saline and bacterial pyrogen incubated in the subject's blood on rectal and oral temperatures and hand blood flow (measured as heat elimination – H.E.) in a human volunteer. The more rapid onset of fever can be seen in the upper panel. (From Gerbrandy *et al.*, 1954a.)

(1954a) found that blood obtained from human subjects and incubated with endotoxin caused, when re-injected into the subject, fever with a much shorter latency of onset than that caused by the same dose of endotoxin injected alone into the same subject (Fig. 3.2). This short latency fever was determined by an interaction of the endotoxin with the leucocyte component of the subject's blood. Grant & Whalen (1953) were able to demonstrate that there appeared to be a fast-acting pyrogen in the blood of rabbits which were treated with typhoid vaccine. Both the rapidly acting pyrogen studied by Gerbrandy *et al.* (1954a) and by Grant & Whalen (1953) could have come from stimulated leucocytes as a new secretion, or could have been an endotoxin moiety coupled to some leucocyte product. The material discovered by Beeson (1948) could not have been altered endotoxin, and much later (Hanson *et al.*, 1980) was shown to be a polypeptide derived from phagocytes originating from bone marrow. It is now clear that the rapidly acting pyrogen found by the other authors is a separate substance and not altered endotoxin. Thus two terms arose for the newly discovered fast-acting pyrogen derived from leucocytes, namely 'leucocyte pyrogen' or 'endogenous pyrogen', and these terms have been used synonymously in the literature since the 1950s. Fessler *et al.* (1961) showed that rabbit leucocytes kept in the cold were not pyrogenic and when disrupted did not release a pyrogen. Similarly, killing the cells by freezing and thawing, heating or keeping them for a long time in the cold prevented their ability to release leucocyte pyrogen. The evidence pointed to the elaboration of the leucocyte pyrogen *de novo* on incubation at 37 °C in saline and that the pyrogen was not present, pre-elaborated and stored in the cells, although more recent work (Lepe-Ziniga & Gery, 1984) found that it, or IL-1 as we now know it, can be stored in monocytes. Interestingly Fessler *et al.* (1961) found that administration of nitrofurazone to the animal donating the leucocytes, or its addition to the incubating medium, blocked the formation of leucocyte pyrogen. This may possibly have been due to protein synthesis inhibition, however, Kaiser & Wood (1962) observed that puromycin does not prevent endogenous pyrogen release, which explanation renders this unlikely. Atkins & Snell (1964) and Snell & Atkins (1965) were able to show that cells from various rabbit tissues were capable of releasing endogenous-type pyrogen. Bodel & Atkins (1967) demonstrated that, of the blood white cells, the monocytes were the most likely source of endogenous pyrogen during incubation with killed bacteria. They demonstrated that blood leukocytes from patients suffering agranulocytosis and acute monocytic leukaemia could liberate endogenous pyrogen when incubated with killed staphylococci. Over the years since then, it has been established that endogenous pyrogen is elaborated by monocytes and by macrophages present in many animal tissues, including human.

The next major problem concerned the chemical nature of endogenous pyrogen(s). There is evidence, gained from experiments performed in the 1960s, that endogenous pyrogen is a protein or polypeptide. However, the problem in its isolation and purification was in the very crude (by modern standards) methods of chemical separation and in the large decrements in pyrogenic activity which occurred with each attempted stage of purification. Murphy *et al.* (1971), in the late Dr Barry Wood's laboratory at Johns Hopkins University, were able to fractionate crude endogenous pyrogen to get an apparently heterogeneous fraction with a pyrogenic activity of about 30 ng protein/1.0 °C fever. Later Dinarello *et al.* (1977) were able to purify a 15–20 kDa endogenous pyrogen fraction (human endogenous pyrogen) to homogeneity, and this fraction was pyrogenic in rabbits in amounts of the order of 2 ng/kg, and the material appeared to be a polypeptide.

The next stage awaited a marriage of the fever scientists with the immunologists. A substance which caused a reduced blood-iron level and stimulated other parts of the acute phase response was found and named leucocyte endogenous mediator or LEM (Kampschmidt, 1978), and another which stimulated T-lymphocytes (lymphocyte activating factor or LAF, was described; Gery & Waksman, 1972). Much work has been done over the last two decades on these and other cytokines, such as cachetin (Saklatvala *et al.*, 1985), which are released in response to challenges of the immune systems. It now turns out that LEM, LAF and leucocyte pyrogen and some others are identical and are the most extensively studied endogenous pyrogen to which the term IL-1 is given. It has a molecular weight of 17.5 kDa (Dinarello, 1988). In fact, though having almost identical biological activities (Dinarello, 1988), IL-1 exists in two biochemically distinct forms namely, IL-1α and IL-1β, and the cDNAs of the two genes which code for them have been cloned (Auron *et al.*, 1984; Lomedico *et al.*, 1984). The IL-1α and β (described more fully below) have many immunological and other functions as well as being pyrogenic. Endotoxins will induce IL-1 production from monocytes or macrophages, but some other exogenous pyrogens do not.

There are now known to be other polypeptide endogenous pyrogens apart from IL-1. One of these is known as IL-6 and formerly known as interferon-β_2. It also may be involved in the whole acute phase response and other aspects of immuno-stimulation.

Interferon-α and interferon-γ, the production of which may be induced both by endotoxins and viruses, are also pyrogenic (Dinarello *et al.*, 1984; Morimoto *et al.*, 1987). Interferon-γ also enhances the production of IL-1 from macrophages. Another endogenous pyrogen, the cytokine known as TNF, acts in part directly as a pyrogen. It has been shown to induce production and release of IL-1 (Dinarello *et al.*, 1986). These four known and chemically distinct polypeptide endogenous pyrogens have different pyrogenic potencies with IL-1 and TNF about equal and the other two rather less potent.

Much of the work on pyrogenic activity of the various cytokines has

been done using injections of these substances either iv or intracerebrally, but the correlation of their circulating blood levels with fever
after administration of bacteria or bacterial pyrogens is still being studied
(Kluger, 1991b), and there is evidence that the circulating levels of
IL-1 do not correlate with the temperature change in fever (Kluger,
1992). Antiserum to recombinant IL-1α was without effect on bacterial
pyrogen-induced fever (Long *et al.*, 1989). Could this be an example of
what T. H. Huxley (1873) called 'the great tragedy of Science – the
slaying of a beautiful hypothesis by an ugly fact', or does it emphasize
that there may be a number of different pyrogenic cytokine pathways
with some cytokines inducing a cascade of mediators some of which we
know and others as yet to be discovered, and with variations depending
on the species studied? Another problem may relate to the assay for IL-1
in different species. Recently a very sensitive radioimmunoassay for
circulating IL-1 has been developed for use in the rat (Derijk &
Berkenbosch, 1992), and using this the authors demonstrated a rise in
the plasma level of IL-1 in response to administration of bacterial
lipopolysaccharide. Even the term IL-1 is not really adequate since there
are at least two forms of IL-1 namely, IL-1α and IL-1β. IL-1α is thought
to be cell-associated and IL-1β is possibly the secreted form of IL-1
(Kluger, 1991a). So IL-1α measured in the circulation might not parallel
the fever response curve but IL-1β would more likely do so. In fact, Long
et al. (1990a,b) showed that antiserum to IL-1β reduced fever caused by
bacterial lipopolysaccharide by 57%. Michie *et al.* (1988) investigated
the plasma levels of several cytokines in healthy human male volunteers
after intravenous administration of bacterial endotoxin. They found that
the plasma level of TNF rose dramatically and roughly paralleled the
fever response but the plasma levels of IL-1β and interferon-γ did not
rise. So here is either a species difference or another paradox. The time
course of the appearance of potentially pyrogenic cytokines in the blood
following administration of bacterial lipopolysaccharide, and their concentrations, have been well discussed by Cannon *et al.* (1992) who make
a case for the increases in plasma IL-1β and IL-6 being due to their
induction by TNFα, and for hepatic macrophages being major sources
of circulating cytokines in endotoxaemia. In the very severe fever of
Plasmodium vivax malaria the plasma levels of TNF were found to rise
and correlate well with the body temperature (Karunaweera *et al.*,
1992), and this adds greatly to the demonstration by Cranston (1959a)
of an endogenous pyrogen in the plasma in malarial fever. Certainly,
antiserum to IL-1β greatly attenuates bacterial pyrogen-induced fever

in the rat (Rothwell 1989) as does an antiserum to TNF in the rabbit (Kawasaki *et al.*, 1989). The plasma and cerebrospinal fluid levels of another cytokine, IL-6, rose in response to injections of IL-1β in a dose-dependent manner and paralleled the rise in core temperature in rats (LeMay *et al.*, 1990). They showed that pre-treatment with an IL-1β antiserum greatly reduced both the fever and the plasma and csf levels of IL-6. This has led to the suggestion that IL-1β fever may be the result of the release of IL-6 induced by IL-1β which is in turn released by bacterial pyrogen. There may be a difficulty in the measurement of some circulating cytokines in that there are soluble cytokine receptors which, in addition to brain and other receptors, can bind the cytokine (Symons & Duff, 1992). If there were an initial very rapid release of IL-1 in response to endotoxin with much of the released cytokine being bound to brain and peripheral receptors within seconds or a few minutes, the timing of blood sampling for assessment could be critical. The initial high level of the cytokine could have been missed. It might be useful to pretreat the animal with an IL-1 receptor blocker and then to give the endotoxin or other exogenous pyrogen since such treatment could unmask the true level of release of IL-1. Dinarello *et al.* (1991) have also demonstrated that IL-6 can not only cause fever on iv administration in the rabbit, but also induces rapid PGE_2 synthesis in the brain, but not in circulating mononuclear cells. A further candidate for the status of endogenous pyrogen is MIP-1 (Davatelis *et al.*, 1989). Another complication is found in the reports that an antiserum to mouse IL-1 did not block bacterial pyrogen fever in the rat and that an antiserum to TNF enhanced fever in the rat (Long *et al.*, 1989, 1990a,b). More work is needed on the *in vivo* responses to these antibodies and on the complex interactions of potentially pyrogenic cytokines. There are two heparin-binding proteins derived from macrophages which are inflammatory: MIP-1 of molecular mass about 8 kDa and MIP-2, of molecular mass about 6 kDa (Wolpe *et al.*, 1989). MIP-1 not only causes a dose-related fever on iv administration, in the rabbit, but the fever is not inhibited by ibuprofen. This suggests that the prostaglandin pathway (see Chapter 5) is not involved in MIP-1 induced fever. MIP-2 does not induce fever in the rabbit.

In consideration of the possible function of a cytokine as an endogenous pyrogen it is useful to use Kluger's (1992) postulates:

1. Application of the substance at a hypothetical locus of action results in the response such as fever observed during infection.

2. When an exogenous factor, e.g. an infecting organism, induces the fever response, the released putative endogenous mediator should be quantitatively related to the magnitude of the response; and the putative endogenous pyrogen should be released in amounts consistent with those needed to cause the response when applied to the locus of its action.
3. Treatment with substances which block the release of the possible mediator should block the fever response.
4. Materials which block the action of the putative mediator should block the response.

So far, most studies of the pyrogenic cytokines released have been made using Gram-negative organisms or their lipopolysaccharide cell wall endotoxins. Some species, for example the baboon (*Papio ursinus*), did not respond to these with fever or indeed exhibit an acute phase response (Zurovsky *et al.*, 1987b). These baboons, however, responded with fever to iv injections of killed *Staphylococcus aureus* (Gram-positive). The rhesus monkey (*Macaca mulatta*) is also reported not to respond to fever when challenged with iv Gram-negative pyrogens except perhaps when very high doses are used (Sheagren *et al.*, 1967), but it does get fever in response to icv Gram-negative endotoxin (Myers *et al.*, 1974). Borsook *et al.* (1978) suggested that the baboon leucocytes might not elaborate IL-1 in response to Gram-negative endotoxin. Another suggestion for the action of another Gram-positive organism inducing fever in the rabbit is that streptococcal pyrogenic exotoxin, at considerable doses, can cross the blood–brain barrier to act directly on the hypothalamus (Schlievert & Watson, 1978). It is possible that some pyrogenic agents could in some species bypass the usual cytokine generation stage. The ubiquity of a febrile response to Gram-negative endotoxins is cast into doubt by the work of Zurovsky *et al.* (1987b) on the baboon, and this stresses the need for great caution in extrapolating from the responses to any one pyrogen or from any one species.

There are neurons within the hypothalamus which can release pyrogenic cytokines, and the possible function of these will be discussed in Chapter 5.

Whether there will be more 'endogenous pyrogens' discovered is open to speculation, but considering the complexity of the pyrogenic and immunological roles of the cytokines so far studied it would be naive to think that there are no more, or that those presently known represent a redundancy in nature's functions in infection and inflammatory disease.

I hope that this chapter gives a sufficient framework for the reader to understand the later chapters in which the main thrust of this book, namely the role of the nervous system in fever, is developed. It is not intended to be a comprehensive survey of the vast field of the study of cytokines and inflammation, infection and fever which in itself would require several volumes to cover. Much of what comes later will deal with the effects of administration of IL-1, TNF, IFNs and endotoxin without further consideration of the peripheral cytokine cascades which might be induced. As will be seen, many of the effects of pyrogenic cytokines have been studied by iv, icv and local micro-injection techniques, and these methods may give indices of how the cytokines *could* act, but do not define necessarily which cytokines are the mediators of fever in specific infections or inflammatory states.

4

The loci of action of endogenous mediators of fever

A careful distinction has to be made between the loci of action in the CNS of endogenous mediators of fever generated by disease processes and the loci revealed by their topical administration for experimental purposes. The techniques for the demonstration of such loci have included the observation of the effects of naturally occurring or experimental lesions, the effects of topical application to various brain regions (by micro-injection perfusion, or micro-dialysis) and the localization of high densities of specific receptors for the fever mediators.

A number of attempts were made in the last century and early in this century to locate regions of the brain responsible for thermoregulation, and then to associate these with the actions of pyrogenic substances. Ott (1887) proposed four 'thermotaxic' regions of the brain namely, the corpus striatum, the tuber cinereum (probably identical to the anterior hypothalamus), and two areas of the cerebral cortex, and Ott in his 1914 lectures proposed these areas as the loci of action of pyrogenic substances. In 1915, Hashimoto injected pyrogens through cannulae into thermosensitive structures in the diencephalon, and found that these injections were more effective than systemic injections of the pyrogens. Likewise, Sheth & Borison (1960) injected salmonella endotoxin into the subarachnoid space or into the cerebral ventricles in cats and dogs and found that fever followed more readily than when the pyrogen was given intravenously. Ranson *et al.* (1939) found that lesions in the posterior and anterior hypothalamus, in cats, reduced or abolished fever caused by systemic injection of typhoid vaccine, but shivering still occurred. The posterior hypothalamic lesions were particularly effective in reducing fever. There is ample evidence for the need for an intact posterior hypothalamus for the development of typical febrile responses to systematically administered pyrogens (Myers, 1969). Chambers *et al.* (1949) attempted to infer the site of action of bacterial pyrogen by lesioning techniques in cats and dogs. Spinal cord transections at the lower cervical and upper thoracic levels prevented fever, but the leucopaenia which follows the iv administration of endotoxin was observed. Decortication left the febrile response intact, but strangely thalamic and caudal hypothalamic lesions did not prevent fever. Decerebration just above the midbrain prevented fever but at the pontile or medullary levels left responses to pyrogens and sometimes caused spontaneous fevers. They concluded that some integrating mechanism was present in the medulla, possibly in the upper spinal cord, which was capable of responding to iv pyrogen by causing fever.

Working with a patient who had suffered a complete spinal cord lesion at C_6–C_7, Cooper *et al.* (1964a) found that intravenous injections of endogenous pyrogen caused marked shivering in the muscles innervated from above the lesion, but not from those innervated from below; and below the lesion there was no skin vasoconstriction, in the hand or fingers. These observations indicate a locus of action of endogenous pyrogen, in the CNS, above the lower cervical level of the spinal cord. These observations confirmed in the human the results of Chambers *et al.* (1949) who, as cited above, found that spinal cord transection in cats and dogs abolished the febrile temperature responses. Perhaps a more important set of observations when considered in the context of the current views of the main locus of action of pyrogenic mediators were the experiments of King & Wood (1958). These experiments showed that blood containing endogenous pyrogen, or the pyrogen derived from sterile white cells, caused fever with a shorter latency and of greater magnitude when injected into the internal carotid artery than it did when given iv. While suggesting an intracranial locus of action of the pyrogen, an action along the course of the brain blood vessels, but outside the brain neuropile, is also a possible interpretation.

The stage was then set for studies of the effects of micro-injection of various pyrogens into the tissue of the brain with greater accuracy because of the availability of better stereotaxic techniques. Villablanca & Myers (1965), micro-injected typhoid vaccine into the hypothalami of cats. They used doses of vaccine ranging from 1/8 to 1/16 000 of that required to produce fever when given intravenously. The vaccine caused fever when given into the anterior hypothalamus or the cerebral ventricles, and the shortest latency to fever was observed with the anterior hypothalamic injections. They concluded that the evidence

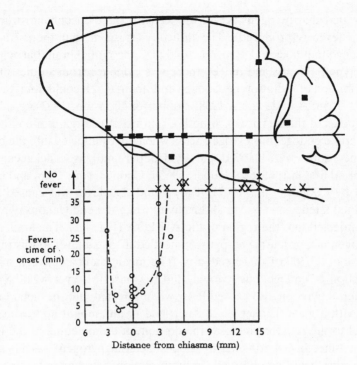

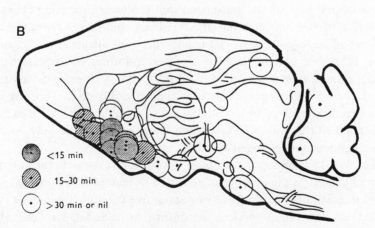

Fig. 4.1. (A) Sagittal section of a rabbit brain 1.5 mm to the right of the mid plane. ■, Site of injection of leucocyte pyrogen; ×, Injection given at ■ and no fever resulted; ○, Time between onset of fever and injection of leucocyte pyrogen in minutes plotted against distance from optic chiasma. (B) Sagittal section of rabbit brain. Centre of circle shows site of injection and circle shows possible limits of spread of leucocyte pyrogen. (From Cooper *et al.*, 1967.)

suggested that pyrogens act on the 'cells of the diencephalic structure when fever is produced'. The difficulty arose in that there was no evidence that bacterial pyrogen could pass the blood–brain barrier into the hypothalamus, and indeed there was evidence from studies of the distribution of radioisotope-labelled endotoxin that it could not (Rowley *et al.*, 1956; Braude *et al.*, 1958; Cooper & Cranston, 1963).

Studies of the loci at which both Gram-negative organism endotoxin and crude endogenous pyrogen acted when micro-injected into the brain of the rabbit were carried out by Cooper and his colleagues, and reported first in 1965–66 (Cooper, 1965b; Cooper *et al.*, 1966) and more fully by Cooper *et al.* (1967). They found that fever was caused with minimal latency and maximal sensitivity when the endogenous pyrogen was injected into the region of the AH/POA (Fig. 4.1). The amount of endogenous, or leucocyte, pyrogen needed to give a fever in this region was about 1/100 of that needed iv. The mean latency between micro-injection of endogenous pyrogen and the onset of fever was 7.8 min. Bacterial pyrogen also caused fever when injected into the same locus, but with a mean latency of 28.8 min and in an amount approximately equal to the required iv dose. In addition, at a time equal to the fever onset time, in experiments in which bacterial pyrogen was injected, leucocytes could be observed (in brain sections) streaming towards the locus of injection. It was postulated that the fever producing effect of bacterial pyrogen injected into the AH/POA could be the result of the release of endogenous pyrogen from white cells attracted to the area. The short but definite latency of fever following the injections of endogenous pyrogen suggested the need for the release of yet another mediator of fever, thought at that time possibly to be one of the monoamines involved in thermoregulation in the region. A conclusion was reached that the AH/POA was a locus, probably the only one, at which endogenous pyrogen could act to cause fever.

In 1967, Jackson reported similar results using cats, with the anterior hypothalamus as the locus most sensitive to endogenous pyrogen, and here the mean latency to fever was about five minutes. Of interest, the injections of typhoid vaccine, in contrast to bacterial pyrogen, were smaller than would be necessary to cause fever on iv injection. In addition, typhoid vaccine also caused fever when injected close to, but outside, the region responding to endogenous pyrogen, and the latter did not cause fever when injected into the preoptic area. Also in 1967, results closely similar to those of Cooper *et al.* (1967) were reported by

Repin & Kratskin (1967) from St. Petersburg (then Leningrad), and their most sensitive region was the medial preoptic area.

Cooper *et al.* (1967) and Repin & Kratskin (1967) used 2 μl injection volumes, and Jackson (1967) used 2–5 μl volumes. These volumes are very large by modern standards, and they leave open the problem of the extent of the diffusion of the injected material. Jackson used the visible diffusion of bromophenol blue to estimate the area of diffusion of endogenous pyrogen. However, there is no evidence that the diffusion distance of the dye follows that of the pyrogen, or that the diffusion of peptides is smooth, i.e., it might be concentrated in concentric spheres like the classical Liesegang rings; and the edge of the dye distribution tells only of the density of dye visible to the human eye and may not be related to the biologically active concentration of the active peptide. So this method, while it may be fortuitously related to pyrogen spread has to be rejected. Cooper *et al.* (1967) used the distance from which leucocytes could be seen moving to the injection site as an index, but although this is a measure of a biological activity it may not define the diffusion in amounts able to cause another biological response, namely, fever. All, however, gave micro-injections round the periphery of the sensitive loci, and finding the region bounded by the loci where the micro-injection does not cause fever seems to be the best way to define the extent of the sensitive area. Thus these early findings could still be relevant in that, should the release of IL-1 from AH/POA neurons be confirmed as part of the events following actions of pyrogenic cytokines outside the brain neuropil, or in response to intracerebral infection, then this locus of action remains confirmed as secondary in the one instance and possibly primary in the other. The use of very large volumes of injected material in the early experiments could have led to its spread to such regions as the OVLT, and certainly could have released prostaglandins in response to the not inconsiderable tissue damage.

Later, Rosendorff & Mooney (1971), using a further purified fraction of leucocyte pyrogen found, in addition to the AH/POA region already described, a locus in the brainstem in the midbrain region which was sensitive to leucocyte pyrogen.

At this time the nature of endogenous pyrogen, other than that it was a low molecular weight protein or peptide, was not known; and no method for labelling pure endogenous pyrogen was known. An earlier attempt to trace the entry of crude endogenous pyrogen into the brain using radioactive labelling was made by Allen (1965). When this labelled material was injected iv, radioactivity was found in the posterior hypothalamus. There is no evidence, however, that the labelled substance or substances were related to the endogenous pyrogen present. Although the weight of evidence showed that micro-injected impure endogenous pyrogen had a maximal pyrogenicity when given into the AH/POA, there was no evidence that the active component could cross the blood–brain barrier. There is evidence from studies using a labelled endogenous pyrogen – cytokine IL-1 – that it does not cross the barrier (Dinarello *et al.*, 1978). So, while the apparent locus of action in the AH/POA at which injected endogenous pyrogen may well be very close to the real site of action of pyrogenic cytokines, there is now evidence that it is not the primary locus of action of blood borne pyrogens. Despite the results of experiments using labelled IL-1 by Dinarello et al. (1978) a more recent study using radio-iodinated IL-1α (Banks *et al.*, 1989) provided evidence for transport of the cytokine into the hypothalamus of the mouse. It appears that there are bi-directional transport systems in the mouse with transport rates far exceeding those predicted for non-specific mechanisms. The AH/POA could still play a direct part in the response to IL-1 from the circulation if indeed this cytokine is the circulating mediator at the blood–brain barrier level, but it could, however, represent an important locus of action of endogenous pyrogens generated by brain infections.

There is also some evidence from experimental lesions that there may be loci other than the AH/POA involved in the induction of fever. Veale & Cooper (1975) made extensive electrolytic lesions of the AH/POA in rabbits and found that they developed fever from iv pyrogen, but not from PGE_1 injected into the lesioned area. Lipton & Trzcinka (1976) found that large lesions in the AH/POA of squirrel monkeys (*Saimiri sciureus*) did not abolish fever caused by *Salmonella typhosa* endotoxin. They were not able to cause fever, however, when the endotoxin was injected into the medullae of the monkeys. They concluded that there is no obligatory role for the AH/POA in the production of fever. Lipton *et al.* (1977) reported a case of a 57-year-old man who had sarcoidosis, who as a result of infiltration into the hypothalamic area had complete 'devastation' of the AH/POA and loss of thermoregulation, but who developed a fever when a massive bed sore became infected. The extent of the hypothalamic damage was verified at autopsy. This is powerful evidence for regions outside the AH/POA being able, in the absence of the AH/POA, to respond to the products of infection by inducing fever. Blatteis & Banet (1986), using microsurgery, interrupted the connections between the preoptic region and the rest of the brainstem in the rat and found only minimal modification of fever, and indeed normal thermoregulation. Such observations do not rule out the AH/POA as a normal participant in the induction of fever in individuals or animals with undamaged brains. Hellon & Townsend (1983) suggested that the ability of animals to get fever in response to systemic administration of pyrogens after AH/POA lesions could be due to the development of, or sensitization of, extra-hypothalamic receptor sites for endogenous pyrogen if the primary receptor sites are destroyed. Cooper & Veale (1972) using rabbits in which the cerebral ventricles had been filled with sterile, pyrogen-free mineral oil, also showed that transport of pyrogens to the AH/POA via the csf was not essential to fever production, and that the csf might be an important route of excretion of pyrogen mediators from the brain since the animals with oil-filled ventricles had much larger and more prolonged fevers than controls. It has been suggested (Bito & Davson, 1974) that prostaglandins, one of which (i.e., $PGE_{2\alpha}$) is a fever mediator, excreted into csf from brain tissue are removed by a carrier system.

The circumventricular organs

New evidence for a locus of action of pyrogenic cytokines outside the brain neuropil, in one or more of the circumventricular organs came to light. Dinarello *et al.*, (1978) studied the distribution of radiolabelled purified human leucocytic pyrogen, in rabbits, and found none in the AH/POA 30 min later even though fever was well developed. This confirmed the earlier evidence by Gander & Milton (1976) who used a less pure pyrogen. This, together with the finding by Lipton *et al.* (1979) that transport inhibitors do not prevent fever developing after intravenous pyrogen injection, led Blatteis *et al.* (1983a), to conclude that the entry of endogenous pyrogen into the brain is likely to be by a process of free diffusion through a region having capillaries without the tight junctions found in most of the brain capillaries. Hellon & Townsend (1983) postulated that the portal of entry of endogenous pyrogen into the hypothalamus might be the OVLT (Fig.4.2). Blatteis *et al.* (1983a) also started to investigate regions where the blood–brain barrier is less tight, such as the circumventricular organs. They made electrolytic lesions in the AV3V in guinea-pigs. Whereas intraperitoneal administration of endotoxin in unoperated or sham operated guinea-pigs caused fever, it did not do so in the animals which had the AV3V

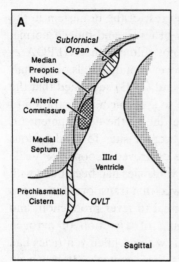
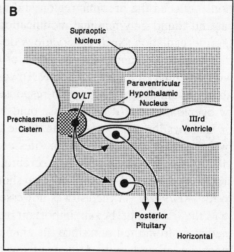

Fig. 4.2. (a) Schematic drawing of a sagittal section of the rat brain illustrating the circumventricular organs. (b) Structure of the organ vasculosum of the lamina terminalis OVLT and its major efferent pathways. (From Johnson & Loewy, 1990.)

lesions. These lesions included the OVLT, an organ having fenestrated capillaries unlike those in the substance of the hypothalamus which have tight junctions, and which is close to the primary site most sensitive to micro-injected pyrogen in the guinea-pig namely the medial preoptic area. He was able to exclude damage to the preoptic area as a cause of the absence of fever in the lesioned animals. Shimada *et al.* (1984), showed that rats which had received iv zymosan, an immunological adjuvant which stimulates RES cells, or which were given iv endotoxin which also stimulates the RES cells, when given iv endogenous pyrogen three days later had markedly enhanced fevers. Stitt *et al.* (1984) also showed that the same enhancement followed injections of minute amounts of these adjuvants into the OVLT. These observations suggested that the OVLT might contain some RES cells, and that it could be a locus of action of endogenous pyrogen. Stitt (1985) made small electrolytic discrete lesions in the OVLT of a size which did not destroy the organ. Three days later fevers in response to iv endogenous pyrogen were enhanced as compared to the fevers obtained before lesioning, and the enhanced fever responses subsided over three weeks. Similar lesions in the AH/POA did not enhance the febrile responses. Two explanations were advanced, namely: (1) the lesions caused increased permeability of the capillaries in the OVLT so that the pyrogen could more easily enter the hypothalamic neuropil or (2) the locally induced inflammatory response sensitized the endogenous pyrogen receptors, possibly by stimulating the local RES cells in a manner similar to the action of zymosan. Thus, there is very good evidence for the OVLT as one locus of action of endogenous pyrogen outside the brain neuropil.

Hashimoto *et al.* (1991), injected IL-1β labelled with colloidal gold into the carotid arteries of pentobarbital sodium anaesthetized rabbits and studied the distribution of the colloidal gold in the forebrains. Electron microscopy showed IL-1-gold conjugates on the surface and in vesicles in the capillaries in the anteroventricular region. In conscious animals the IL-1-gold conjugates caused fever when given intravenously, whereas colloidal gold alone did not. The location of the gold accumulation provides evidence for a region close to the OVLT, but not necessarily within, as a locus in which IL-1β receptors would be expected to exist. Further studies of IL-1 binding sites are under way at the time of writing, and these together with local sites of action of the recently available IL-1 receptor blocker should add further evidence on this matter.

The evidence for the role of the OVLT was strengthened by Blatteis *et al.* (1987), who made discrete lesions in the AV3V regions in sheep. In the sheep the rostral wall of the third ventricle contains an elongated OVLT enabling lesions to be made which separate off regions of that organ. Fever was reduced by medial lesions going from the floor of the third ventricle to the anterior commissure, and which extended laterally into periventricular preoptic tissue. Lesions which did not include the base of the OVLT did not alter the febrile response to iv pyrogens nor did lesions of the lateral wall of the third ventricle or of the AH/POA provided that the anterior wall of the ventricle was left intact.

Further evidence for the OVLT as an important locus of action of endogenous pyrogens comes from experiments in which TNF increased the firing rates of 44% of OVLT neurons in guinea-pig brain slices (Shibata & Blatteis, 1991b). Nakamori *et al.* (1993) studied IL-1β production in the rabbit brain in response to intravenous endotoxin using *in situ* hybridization and immuno-histochemistry. IL-1β production was not observed at an endotoxin dose of $0.02\,\mu g.kg^{-1}$, but at $4\,\mu g.kg^{-1}$ it was seen to occur in the OVLT, and was located to macrophages. At 10 times the dose of endotoxin there was widespread non-specific IL-1β in many brain areas. They postulate that the OVLT IL-1β production might be related to the second peak of fever seen with moderately high doses of endotoxin.

The use of colchicine to produce reversible lesions in or near the OVLT has been used in the study of water and electrolyte balance (Thornton *et al.*, 1987). It would seem that this technique could be of use in longitudinal studies of the effect of altered OVLT function, and possibly of pathways from it, on pyrogen-induced fever.

If it can be safely assumed that the release of PGE$_2$ into the hypothalamic neuropil is one important step in the genesis of fever, it could be postulated that such release might take place within, or in regions adjacent to, the OVLT. This could be one mechanism of transduction of the action of endogenous pyrogens into signals to the thermoregulatory control neuron pools. Using tritium labelled PGE$_2$, Matsumura *et al.* (1990) found a high density of PGE$_2$ binding in the anterior wall of the third ventricle, close to the ventricle and surrounding the OVLT; but there was very little within the OVLT. Using micro-dialysis techniques, Komaki *et al.* (1992) showed that IL-1β injected intravenously in the rabbit caused rapid release of PGE$_2$ into the interstitial fluid of the OVLT and the medial preoptic area, and release occurred much later in other hypothalamic areas. The rapid response was inhibited by indomethacin.

Shibata & Blatteis (1991a) found that TNF and IFNs increased the firing rate of single units within the OVLT, measured using extracellular electrodes. Of the units studied 44% had raised firing rates and 56% did not. The increase in firing rate lasted 30.6–57.5 min (mean 47.4). This result is consistent with the OVLT being a site in which the circulating cytokine signals could be transduced into neuronal activity, signalling further possibly to the thermoregulatory apparatus.

Knowing that the calcium channel blocking agent verapamil given iv reduces the fever induced by iv endogenous pyrogen, and that it is without effect on the fever caused by injecting PGE into the OVLT, Stitt & Shimada (1991) injected verapamil into the OVLT and assessed its effect on fever caused by endogenous pyrogen. It greatly reduced the fever. Verapamil injected into the OVLT in the absence of a pyrogen had no effect on the rats' core temperatures. The dose of verapamil needed to attenuate fever when given into the OVLT was less than 1/250 of that needed iv. The drug had no effect on the fever consequent on the micro-injection of PGE into the OVLT. The evidence suggested that the calcium channel blocker blocks fever by acting within the OVLT rather than acting peripherally, and that PGE in that region does not induce fever by acting as a calcium ionophore.

Injections into the OVLT could cause artifactual responses if the osmolarity of the injected material is not carefully controlled. Nissen *et al.* (1993) have found that the membrane depolarization, which occurred in some OVLT neurons, was in response to raising the osmotic pressure in the fluid superfusing the explant. This is not surprising in view of the osmoregulatory role of the OVLT. Whether the neurons that respond to febrogenic cytokines would respond in a similar way, or would be influenced by the other neurons which do, is yet to be determined, but these reported observations emphasize the need for very careful examinations of all aspects of the composition of materials injected into the region of the OVLT.

The evidence that IL-1 is capable within the OVLT of inducing fever is strong. It would be reasonable to postulate that the OVLT could also be the main locus of action of other pyrogenic cytokines, e.g., IL-6, TNF and IFNs. We await more definitive studies concerning the distribution of receptors for these substances in the CNS.

Other circumventricular organs and possibly the pineal organ would merit further study, at least to exclude them as sites of pyrogen action. Riedel (1990) has postulated a lower brainstem locus of action of pyrogens from which excited neurons in the long ascending 5-HT containing pathways to the raphe nuclei and above could cause or modify fever. A possible action could be activation of some specific part of the general arousal system with an alteration in gain of the cold defence mechanisms. This is speculative but worth a follow up. Morimoto *et al.* (1988), suggested that prostaglandins synthesized outside the blood–brain barrier could act at multiple sites in the CNS to induce the first phase of fever, and that the second phase of a biphasic fever could result from the action of endogenous pyrogens at the OVLT where the prostaglandin mediator is released.

Other circumventricular organs include the subfornical organ, the area postrema and the median eminence. The subfornical organ is found in the roof of the third ventricle, the area postrema is at the caudal end of the fourth ventricle and the median eminence lies in the floor of the fourth ventricle. These areas also have specialized fenestrated capillaries, providing special properties for exchange across the blood–brain barrier.

Of possible sites of entry of endogenous pyrogens into the brain, the work of Takahashi *et al.* (1993) makes it unlikely that the subfornical organ is one, since lesioning it did not alter the magnitude of fever. Recent preliminary work by Pittman *et al.* (1994, personal communication) found that lesions in the region of the area postrema reduced the fever in some, but not all, rats in response to systemic administration of pyrogen. This suggests that the area postrema should be further examined and, if the initial observations could be confirmed, it might be shown to be another locus of action of pyrogens. It is of particular interest since lesions of the OVLT made in rats do not appear to prevent or alter fever in response to circulating pyrogens (Pittman, 1994, personal communication). Again, if these results can be confirmed they would underline the need for a more extensive study of the role of the OVLT in fever in a wider variety of species some of which may use different circumventricular regions as the loci of action of pyrogens on the brain. It also emphasizes the difficulties frequently encountered by our tendency to extrapolate from the responses seen in only a few species to the creation of universal hypotheses!

Sirko *et al.* (1989) found PGE release in the posterior hypothalamic/tuberal region in response to systemic IL-1 or endotoxin administration in cats. That PGE is released in this region might suggest yet another locus of action of endogenous pyrogen which could possibly penetrate the neuropil. The function of this PGE release into the tuberal region is unknown. It could be that afferent neurons from these regions could be stimulated to have an effect on the hypothalamic thermoregulator as part of the thermoregulation system, or there could be stimulation of part of the arousal systems which could modulate the thermoregulatory set point. These comments on the findings of Sirko *et al.* (1989) are, of course, entirely speculative.

It is also important to realize that the circumventricular organs subserve many functions including neuroendocrine control, osmo-regulation and the regulation of body water to mention but a few. Some of these are also of importance in fever and the acute phase reaction, since water balance may be compromised in severe fevers, and the neuroendocrine axis is a part of the neuro-immunological management. Our tendency to consider only the function in which we are mainly interested to the exclusion of other functions controlled via the same region often detracts from our ability to consider important integrated body functions.

The aspects of the acute phase response other than fever, include changes in plasma levels of trace metals such as iron, copper and zinc, and alterations in circulating immunoproteins. The locus of action of endogenous pyrogen and PGE in the initiation of these changes was studied by Blatteis *et al*. (1983b). They concluded that both fever and the non-febrile aspects of the acute phase response were mediated via the preoptic region, and that the prostaglandin was involved only in mediating fever. Sakata *et al*. (1993) stimulated the region near the AH/POA and found that the acute phase response (non-febrile) was not induced, and electrical stimulation of the AV3V if anything initiated responses opposite to those seen after preoptic stimulation. They concluded that non-specific stimulation of the preoptic region did not cause the non-febrile acute phase responses. Thus the results of Blatteis *et al*. (1983b) were likely to have been specific responses to endogenous pyrogen.

5

Beyond the loci of action of circulating pyrogens: mediators and mechanisms

Distribution and actions of first signal transducers of fever within the brain

α-Prostaglandins – actions, enzymes, location and receptors

Prostaglandins are highly biologically active substances derived from polyunsaturated fatty acids. Those of particular concern to us in the study of fever are derivatives of arachidonic acid the structural formula of which is given in Fig. 5.1. Arachidonic acid is released from the phospholipids in cell membranes by the action of phospholipases and other lipases. A pathway from arachidonic acid to PGE_2 using cyclo-oxygenase, peroxidase and PGE_2 isomerase is given in Fig. 5.2. A closely similar prostaglandin, which induces febrile responses, is PGE_1, the structural formula of PGE_2 is shown in Fig. 5.3.

The immense amount of work on the role of prostaglandins on the CNS mediation of fever began with the observations of Milton & Wendlandt (1970). They injected endotoxin into the lateral cerebral ventricles of cats and observed that the resulting fever was prevented by the drug 4-acetamidophenol, a known antipyretic. Seeking to identify a substance or substances which might act as mediators of fever in the CNS, and which might be excreted into the csf, they noted something which had biological activity when tested on the rat stomach fundus strip, but they did not have sufficient material for its identification. Astutely realizing that the rat fundus strip was known to respond in a similar way to PGE_1, they tried injecting microgram amounts of PGE_1 into the cat's lateral cerebral ventricle and found that it caused a typical fever. This was reported in Milton & Wendlandt (1970) along with the interesting finding that 4-acetoamidophenol did not block the fever caused by intraventricularly administered PGE_1. They suggested that

60

COOH
arachidonic acid

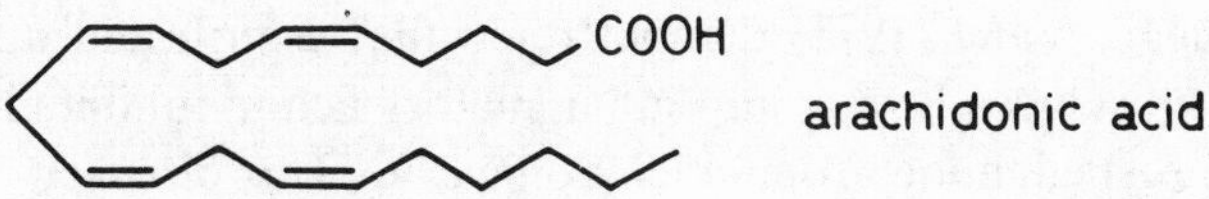

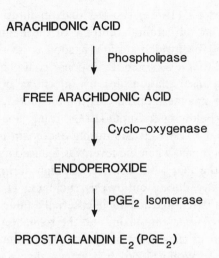

Fig. 5.1. Structure of arachidonic acid.

ARACHIDONIC ACID
Phospholipase
FREE ARACHIDONIC ACID
Cyclo-oxygenase
ENDOPEROXIDE
PGE2 Isomerase
PROSTAGLANDIN E2 (PGE2)

Fig. 5.2. The pathway from arachidonic acid to PGE_2.

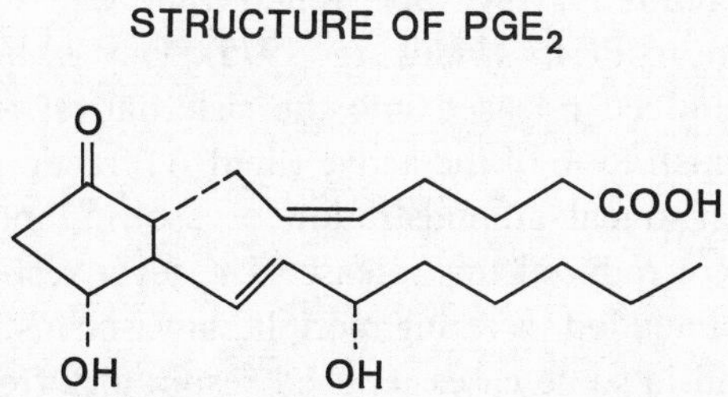

STRUCTURE OF PGE2
O
COOH
OH
OH

Fig. 5.3. Structure of PGE_2.

PGE_1 might act to modulate body temperature and that the antipyretic action could be to prevent PGE_1 being released by pyrogen. Later, Milton & Wendlandt (1971) showed a good dose relationship between the extent of fever and the intraventricular dose of PGE_1 in the 10 ng to 1 μg range. Vane (1971) demonstrated that aspirin and other non-steroidal substances having anti-inflammatory action inhibited the synthesis of prostaglandins from arachidonic acid. This discovery together with the observations of Milton & Wendlandt (1970) opened up a new field in the understanding of the CNS action of pyrogens and antipyretics.

Feldberg & Saxena (1971a) showed that an infusion of PGE_1 at 20 ng/min into a lateral cerebral ventricle of the unanaesthetized cat caused a prolonged fever which subsided as soon as the infusion stopped. They also showed that a good febrile response could be obtained (with a clear dose response relationship) by injections of PGE_1, in the 2–100 ng range in unanaesthetized cats, rabbits and rats (Feldberg & Saxena 1971a,b). Feldberg & Gupta (1973), using bioassays on the rat fundus examined the vcsf collected during endotoxin induced fever in the cat and also obtained when the fever was reduced by an antipyretic. They found that the PGE_1-like activity was high during the fever and was reduced greatly during antipyresis. Feldberg *et al.* (1973) also showed the rise in PGE_1-like activity in cisternal csf during fever caused by iv *Shigella dysenteriae* endotoxin, and the reduction in that activity during the antipyresis caused by intraperitoneal indomethacin.

Since Coceani & Wolfe (1966) had shown that several groups of prostaglandins can contract the rat fundus preparation, and having excluded by thin layer chromatography the F prostaglandins, Feldberg sent samples of his cat csf, obtained during fever, to Dr. Heather Davis for radioimmunoassay. She found that the activity was almost entirely due to PGE_2 (Feldberg, 1975). Dey *et al.* (1975) found that PGE_2 was indeed released into the cisternal csf following intraventricular administration of the active (lipid A) fraction of endotoxin, and that intraperitoneal administration of aspirin, indomethacin or 4-acetamidophenol reduced this release. The fever responses to intraventricular PGE included shivering, peripheral vasoconstriction, curling up into a ball and in some cases reduced respiratory frequency.

Studies were then undertaken to compare the loci at which PGE_1 or PGE_2 injected into the substance of the brain would cause fever, and to compare these with the loci at which IL-1, similarly administered, caused fever. Veale & Cooper (1975) micro-injected PGE_1 into the AH/POA, the lateral hypothalamus, the midbrain, the hippocampus and the amygdala. They used doses ranging from 0.1 ng to 50 ng at each site. The only region responding to the PGE_1 injection with fever, other than to the largest (50 ng) dose, was the AH/POA. The large dose also caused fever in some experiments when given into the lateral hypothalamus, and this could have been due to diffusion to the AH/POA. They noted that as little as 100 pg of PGE_1 injected into the AH/POA could cause fever. Perhaps the most extensive mapping of PGE_1 sensitive sites in the rat brain is that of Williams *et al.* (1977). There was remarkable correspondence between the loci at which the prostaglandin caused fever at 50 ng and 100 ng doses and the previously demonstrated loci at which micro-injections of endogenous pyrogens caused fever. It is interesting also to note that they found a few loci, e.g., in the posterior hypothalamus/tuberal region at which 100 ng doses of PGE_1 injections caused fever, and these loci had access to csf spaces. Stitt (1973) had also demonstrated that the anterior hypothalamus of the rabbit responded to micro-injections of PGE_1 in a dose dependent manner, over the range of 20 ng to 1000 ng, with fever. He did not observe fever in response to micro-injection of the prostaglandin into the posterior hypothalamus or the midbrain reticular formation. He also made two very important additional observations namely, (1) that when the anterior hypothalamus was heated during the fevers they were attenuated and that when it was cooled the fevers were exaggerated, and thus the hypothalamic thermosensitivity was retained during the fevers, and (2) that the mechanism of fever production, e.g., augmented heat production or peripheral vasoconstriction depended on the environmental temperature.

With the recent evidence that the OVLT may be the primary locus of action of extra-cranially generated pyrogenic cytokines, the possibility that the initial site of PGE release and action is there, also demands consideration. Stitt (1991) has shown that the OVLT is exquisitely sensitive to PGE_2 in the generation of fever. Fig. 5.4, taken from Stitt (1986), shows fever dose response relationships for PGE_2 in different areas of the rat brain. The lowest threshold was in the OVLT ~0.2 ng versus 1 ng for the AH/POA or the rostral third ventricle, and it appears as though the slope of the relationship also is greater in the OVLT. Several studies have been made of the localization of PGE_2 in both monkey and rat brains. Watanabe *et al.* (1988) investigated the binding sites of several prostaglandins in the monkey brain using [H³] labelled compounds and found sites in many parts of the brain. There was a high density of binding sites in the medial preoptic area and paraventricular nuclei, many in the hypothalamus especially in the supramamillary nuclei, and numerous sites in the thalamus. Matsumura *et al.* (1992), in a study of the rat brain found a similar distribution of PGE_2 binding sites

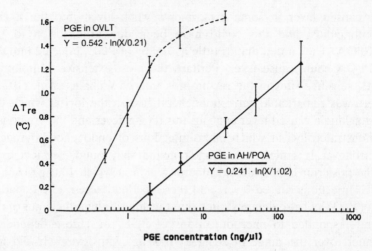

Fig. 5.4. A comparison of the fever dose-response curves to PGE in rats when the PGE is micro-injected into either the AH/POA or the OVLT region. Each curve is composed from the data derived from groups of eight rats, and the slope and intercept of the linear portion of each curve was derived by regression analysis. A comparison of both the slope and the dose threshold of the two equations indicates that the OVLT region is much more sensitive than the AH/POA in the production of fever by PGE. (From Stitt, 1986.)

with particularly dense concentrations in the anterior third ventricle (close to the OVLT), the thalamus, the pontine parabrachial nucleus and the nucleus of the tractus solitarius. The high density of PGE_2 binding sites in the anterior wall of the third ventricle has been observed, using quantitative autoradiography of $[H^3]PGE_2$. Binding sites have also been found in the cerebral cortex, the hippocampus, the septal areas, the BST, the amygdala, the hypothalamic nuclei, the thalamus and the mesencephalon. Fuller details are given in Table 5.1, taken from Matsumura *et al.* (1992). Using an immunoreactivity staining technique, Fujimoto *et al.* (1992) demonstrated the distribution of a tightly bound form of PGE_2 in the rat brain. Again, there was a wide distribution in the brain with particularly high concentrations in parts of the cerebral cortex, the hypothalamic paraventricular nuclei and parts of the midbrain, pons, medulla and cerebellum.

Others have studied the distribution of the enzymes (cyclo-oxygenase and endoperoxide synthase) in the brains of monkeys and sheep. The distribution of endoperoxide synthase in the monkey brain is shown in Table 5.2, taken from Tsubokura *et al.* (1991). The distribution can be seen to be mostly in neurons which are widely spread throughout the brain. In another study, Breder *et al.* (1992) showed cyclo-oxygenase immunoreactivity in many parts of the CNS in neuronal cell bodies and dendrites. The highest abundances were found in forebrain sites including the cerebral cortex, the hippocampus, the amygdala, the BST, the OVLT and in parts of the hypothalamus. While the distributions of these enzymes roughly parallel the PGE_2 binding sites, there is not complete correlation. The relative ubiquity of the PGE_2 distribution in the brain may emphasize the many possible functional roles for the substance, including those subserving autonomic functions; and should the action of fever-inducing cytokines release PGE_2 from many or all of these sites, the levels of PGE_2 in vcsf would be difficult to correlate with that released from any one site. That there is evidence for numerous PGE_2 binding sites in the region of the OVLT, but not within the OVLT, adds weight to the hypothesis that IL-1 acting on the OVLT can trigger PGE release from neurons projecting to the thermoregulatory regions of the hypothalamus. The current wisdom is that PGE_2 acts presynaptically but not as a neurotransmitter. Again the sensitivity of the AH/POA to prostaglandins in causing fever may be in part due to leaking of these substances, when micro-injected, to the vicinity of the OVLT as well as a primary action in the AH/POA itself. In all instances in which PGE_1 or PGE_2 act in the AH/POA or OVLT to cause fever, the onset of the fever process is immediate as compared to the significant delay when IL-1 or cruder endogenous pyrogen preparations are injected into the same regions.

Another important study (Komaki *et al.*, 1992), was undertaken in which recombinant human IL-1 was given intravenously to rats and micro-dialysis probes, perfused with artificial csf, were placed in various regions of the brain. The IL-1 induced rapid release of PGE_2 into the dialysis fluid when the probe was in the OVLT and the medial part of the medial preoptic area. This release was greater and faster than in any other brain area. Indomethacin in the perfusate prevented the appearance of PGE_2 in the perfusing fluid. This is powerful evidence for the OVLT as a major locus of PGE_2 release in response to a circulating pyrogenic cytokine.

Rotondo *et al.* (1988) observed raised PGE_2 levels in the blood throughout fever caused by three pyrogenic agents used: Poly I:Poly C, endotoxin and endogenous pyrogen. The PGE_2 plasma levels rose six to eight fold during fever. If the animal was given ketoprofen during fever both the core temperature and the PGE_2 level in the plasma fell concurrently, but if the rabbit was pre-treated with ketoprofen neither

Table 5.1. *Density of PGE$_2$ binding sites in rats brain (mean and SD)*

	Mean (fmol/mg tissue)	SD
Telencephalon		
Retrosplenial cortex	1.8	0.67
Piriform cortex	2.1	0.29
Temporal cortex	2.1	0.99
Occipital cortex	1.1	0.36
Entorhinal cortex	5.5	0.34
Cingulate cortex	1.8	0.21
Hippocampus (dorsal-lateral)	1.1	0.38
Hippocampus (ventral)	6.2	0.86
Caudate putamen	1.6	0.59
Medial septum	2.2	1.49
Lateral septum	2.3	0.61
Diagonal band of Broca	1.4	0.46
Accumbens nucl.	1.7	0.58
Bed nucleus stria terminalis	4.0	1.13
Amygdala (cortical part)	5.2	1.39
Amygdala (other parts)	2.9	0.67
Diencephalon		
a3v	15.9	0.63
Preoptic area (medial)	2.8	0.45
Preoptic area (lateral)	1.9	0.32
Hypothalamus (anterior)	3.0	0.32
Hypothalamus (lateral)	2.2	0.67
Hypothalamus (ventromedial)	2.8	0.30
Hypothalamus (dorsomedial)	9.4	2.60
Hypothalamus (posterior)	3.0	0.18
Hypothalamus (mammillary)	9.3	2.23
Thalamus (central medial)	7.9	1.24
Thalamus (mediodorsal)	2.2	0.26
Thalamus (laterodorsal/lateropost.)	7.1	0.95
Thalamus (paraventricular)	10.7	0.92
Thalamus (ventral)	1.6	0.78
Thalamus (rhomboid/reuniens)	8.4	0.46
Thalamus (anteroventral)	10.2	2.45
Thalamus (posterior)	1.6	0.56
Thalamus (lateral geniculate)	1.2	0.50
Lateral habenula	1.6	0.75
Medial habenula	2.5	0.42
Mesencephalon		
Interpeduncular nucl.	2.0	1.10
Substantia nigra	1.0	0.49
Central grey	7.7	0.75
Superior colliculus	5.9	0.31
Pons and medulla oblongata		
Motor nucl. 3	1.7	0.57

Table 5.1. *contd.*

	Mean (fmol/mg tissue)	SD
Motor nucl. 7	1.6	0.19
Motor nucl. 5	1.1	0.44
Parabrachial nucl. (dorsal)	12.9	2.89
Raphe magnus	1.9	0.80
Raphe pallidus	6.6	1.50
Raphe obscurus	5.1	0.58
Raphe dorsalis	4.9	1.20
Raphe medialis	1.0	0.27
Reticular form. (gigant)	1.1	0.20
Reticular form. (lateral)	1.0	0.59
Inferior olive	1.1	0.52
Hypoglossal nucl.	1.5	0.29
Nucl. solitary tract (medial)	17.3	1.81
Dorsal motor vagal nucl.	5.3	0.94
Area postrema	1.8	0.77
Locus coeruleus	7.3	0.53
Spinal trig. nucl. (marginal layer)	7.0	1.28
Spinal cord (laminae 1 and 2)	5.8	0.39

(From Matsumura *et al.*, 1992.)

the body temperature nor the PGE_2 plasma level rose. Non-febrile hyperthermia did not induce a rise in plasma prostaglandin. These observations have led to one hypothesis, namely, that the source of the prostaglandin in fever is peripheral, with possibly an entry into the relevant neuropil via the OVLT. In experiments reported by Dascombe (1986) PGE_2 infused into the carotid artery in the rabbit did not raise the body temperature neither did arachidonic acid. Also, in rabbits treated with endotoxin to loosen the blood–brain barrier intra-arterial PGE_2 did not cause fever whereas given into the brain it did. These observations are not consistent with a peripheral source of PGE_2 as the main, or sole, inducer of fever unless it is assumed that the peripheral release of PGE_2 is at the surface or within the OVLT or other possible loci of pyrogen action. As Coceani (1991) has pointed out, the fact that cyclo-oxygenase inhibitors administered into the cerebral ventricles inhibit fever due to systemic administration of pyrogen, argues against a dominant role for the peripheral PGE_2 production in endotoxin fever. Of course the peripheral PGE production could result in a secondary PGE release in the AH/POA which could then be blocked by intra-ventricular administration of a cyclo-oxygenase inhibitor. There is

Table 5.2. *Percentage of positive cells and relative intensity of PES-immunoreactivity in monkey brain regions*

		Nerve cell		Glial cell	
		%	Intensity	%	Intensity
Frontal cortex	I	23	+	22	+
	II	100	+++	19	+
	III	95	++	13	+
	IV	100	++	11	+
	V	97	++	10	+
	VI	100	++	11	+
	W*	—	—	54	+
Temporal cortex	I	13	+	22	++
	II	100	+++	7	+
	III	100	++	5	+
	IV	100	++	22	+
	V	100	++	14	+
	VI	100	++	7	+
	W*	—	—	48	+
Parietal cortex	I	20	+	46	+
	II	100	+++	18	+
	III	100	++	8	+
	IV	100	++	11	+
	V	100	++	10	+
	VI	100	++	19	+
	W*	—	—	41	+
Occipital cortex	I	14	+	18	+
	II	100	+++	8	+
	III	100	++	5	+
	IV	99	++	12	+
	V	100	++	10	+
	VI	99	++	10	+
	W*	—	—	50	+
Globus pallidus		20	++	11	+
Putamen		65	++	19	+
Caudate		92	++	28	+
Amygdala		78	++	17	+
Thalamus		75	++	30	+
Hypothalamus		100	+++	15	+
Hippocampus granular cell layer					
CA4		92	+++	21	+
CA3		87	+++	30	+
CA2		84	+++	17	+
CA1		80	+++	29	+
dentate gyrus		100	+++	nd	+
Cerebullum molecular layer					
molecular layer		40	+	44	+

Table 5.2. *contd.*

	Nerve cell		Glial cell	
	%	Intensity	%	Intensity
Purkinje cell layer	63	+	nd	
granular layer	100	+	nd	
W*	—	−	67	+
Pons	41	+	13	+
Medulla oblongata	74	+	33	+
Spinal cord	63	+	76	+

The population of immunoreactive cells from more than 300 cells, good-shaped (avoided from the counting error because of the irregular sectioning), in each structure were counted under light microscope, and relative intensity of immunoreactivity was graded from + (weak) to +++ (intense).
*White matter; nd: not detected.
(From Tsubokura *et al.*, 1991.)

evidence that in the guinea-pig there may be release of PGE_2 into the preoptic interstitial fluid in endotoxin fever, and that this release could be dissociated from fever (Székely *et al.*, 1994). The role of PGE_2 in fever is assessed below, but it is far from simple.

At this stage we can sum up the evidence that PGE_2 is a major factor in the fevers due to the action of peripheral pyrogens:

1. PGE can be detected in csf and in tissue perfusates from regions of the brain which respond to the pyrogenic cytokines.
2. The regions in which pyrogens generate fever respond to minute amounts of the prostaglandin to cause fever.
3. The administration of substances which block the enzymatic pathways necessary for the prostaglandin synthesis, abolish or greatly attenuate fever.
4. The febrogenic response to topically applied PGEs occurs in *almost* all species so far tested.
5. The onset of fever when the PGEs are micro-injected into the AH/POA or OVLT is almost instantaneous.
6. There are binding sites for PGE_2 close to the OVLT, a probable locus of action of pyrogenic cytokines.
7. There are enzyme systems for the synthesis of PGE_2 in or close to the putative sites of action of the prostaglandin.

These arguments have been well reviewed and extended recently (Coceani, 1991). The proposed action of PGE_2 as a mediator of fever has been made more complicated by two further observations. Morimoto *et al.* (1988), micro-injected PGD_2, PGE_2 and $PGF_{2\alpha}$ into many brain areas as well as into the third cerebral ventricle. They found that PGE_2 and $PGF_{2\alpha}$ induced fever when given into the ventricle in doses of 100 to 1000 ng. Tissue injections in amounts less than 200 ng of PGE_2 and $PGF_{2\alpha}$ into the nucleus Broca ventralis, the AH/POA and ventromedial hypothalamus also caused fever. Other regions only responded with fever if very large doses of the prostaglandins were given, and this makes the interpretation of the responses difficult. PGD_2 did not seem to have a pyrogenic role. In the first peak of biphasic fever prostaglandin synthesized outside the blood–brain barrier seemed to act on multiple brain sites, and in the second peak, endogenous pyrogen acts near the OVLT to release PGE.

β-*Prostaglandins – a sole or obligatory role as a fever mediator?*

While there is evidence that PGE_2 can play an important role as a brain mediator of fever, there are also arguments that it may not be the sole or even an obligatory mediator. There is considerable agreement that the prostaglandin may have an important role in the initial stage of fever, and that there may be other arachidonic acid derived pyrogens (Laburn *et al.*, 1977; Székely & Komaromi, 1978). Morimoto *et al.* (1987), have postulated that prostanoids contribute to two phases of fever, the one being the first part of a biphasic fever induced by action of prostanoids synthesized outside the brain and the second phase mediated by their synthesis within the brain.

The main arguments against a sole action of PGE_2 as the final mediator of endotoxin induced and other fevers are as follows (see Mitchell *et al.*, 1986). The first is the lack of fever in *some* species, e.g., newborn lambs and goats, in response to intraventricular PGE even though intravenous endotoxin caused fever. Then, in rabbits, it is possible to suppress the rise in csf PGE levels with salicylate or indomethacin but still retain the normal fever response to endogenous pyrogen. But, the PGE present in csf may come from many parts of the CNS and there may well not be a good correlation with that produced solely in the thermoregulatory regions. Again, the possibility of protein binding of PGE in the csf makes interpretation of the measurable PGE levels more difficult. The tissue concentrations of micro-injected PGE necessary to cause fever, when calculated from the injected dose, are much higher than is likely to occur in systemically induced fever thus making the interpretation of micro-injection experiments difficult. Cranston *et al.* (1976a,b) have given icv injections of two prostaglandin antagonists to rabbits which prevented fever developing after icv injections of PGE_2 but did not alter fever brought on by endogenous pyrogen. Ablation of the AH/POA (Veale & Cooper, 1975) prevented fever due to icv or AH/POA tissue injection of PGE but did not stop the fever induced by intravenous endogenous pyrogen, though that fever was of slower onset. If changes in the firing rates of hypothalamic thermosensitive units are indeed related to the development of fever then the inconsistency of the effects of PGE on them as compared to the consistent and logical response to endogenous pyrogens is difficult to reconcile with an action of PGE in causing fever (see page 76). Such arguments do not rule out a role for PGE in the development of fever, especially in the rapid onset phase, but they do point to the possibility that there may be other non-prostanoid pathways available. Scott *et al.* (1987) measured the release of PGE_2 caused by leucocyte pyrogen in guinea-pig hypothalamic slices and found a dose related release. However, the tissue levels were much lower than those required to cause fever by micro-injection, and this suggested perhaps that another mediator was necessary.

Cranston *et al.* (1980) have found that fever induced by endogenous pyrogen in the rabbit was suppressed by icv administration of anisomycin, which is a protein synthesis inhibitor. They (Cranston *et al.*, 1982) also found that the dose response curves for anisomycin/fever relationship and anisomycin/[14]leucine incorporation into hypothalamic protein were similar. This finding agrees with that of Siegert *et al.* (1976) who, using another protein synthesis inhibitor – cyclohexamide – found that this compound suppressed endogenous pyrogen induced fever. The nature of the protein synthesis which is inhibited is not known, but it could be in part the elaboration of enzymes necessary for prostaglandin synthesis, IL-1 in hypothalamic neurons or a protein mediator of fever not yet discovered.

From the OVLT to the AH/POA and beyond

If we accept, as a working hypothesis, that the elaboration of PGE_2 is induced by pyrogenic cytokines in or near the OVLT, the next stage is to establish the connection between this event and the alteration in thermoregulation which causes fever. A theoretical model for part of this connectivity is shown in Fig. 5.5 (taken from Coceani, 1991), and another from Stitt (1986) is shown in Fig. 5.6. In this the IL-1 interaction with its receptor either activates a link to a neuron which terminates in the anterior hypothalamus where it in turn induces the release of PGE_2 in that region, or that the IL-1 interaction with its receptor enables the stimulation of local reticuloendothelial cells to release PGE_2 which diffuses into the anterior hypothalamus, or both. PGE_2 from the circulation could also diffuse from the OVLT to reach the hypothalamus. A similar schema is given by Murakami (1992) who also suggested that IL-1β could, in the rabbit, diffuse from the OVLT into the brain interstitium and there release arachidonate metabolites other than PGE_2. The schema was drawn up to explain the findings that iv indomethacin attenuated both peaks of fever, but icv indomethacin blocked only the second peak of fever. This latter action was proposed to account for the second component of a biphasic fever. It is interesting to note that both IL-1 and IL-6 have been shown to release PGE_2, and only this prostaglandin, in hypothalamic explants (Navarra *et al.*, 1992). There are reports of neurons in the hypothalamus that contain IL-1 immunoreactive material (Breder *et al.*, 1988), and there are IL-1 receptors there also (Farrar *et al.*, 1987). There is also TNF reactive material in the mouse hypothalamus (Breder & Saper, 1988). One hypothesis which has been proposed is that PGE_2 from the OVLT, or OVLT neurons stimulated by PGE_2, could induce secondary release of IL-1 in the hypothalamus leading to further release locally of prostaglandins. Alternatively, infection or inflammation within the brain could evoke a similar response. Saper & Breder (1992) have used enzyme assays, immunocytochemistry and immunoblotting to locate neurons in regions of the brain thought to play a part in the local secretion of prostaglandins, and the components of the febrile response. Their observations support an hypothesis that circulating pyrogenic cytokines could act within the OVLT to release PGE_2 which would diffuse to the AH/POA, there to act on cytokine containing neurons, and also through them, to release further cytokines more distally to evoke the autonomic endocrine and behavioural changes of fever. So that if more evidence confirms that peripheral pyrogens can cause secondary release of either IL-1 or IL-6 in the hypothalamus, and elsewhere in the fever pathway, a more convincing mechanism for them to cause fever can be postulated. Some evidence for a role of IL-1 released in the brain has been provided by Fontana *et al.* (1984) who injected mice intraperitoneally with

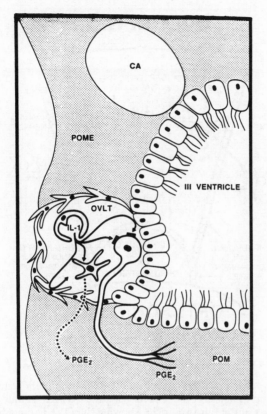

Fig. 5.5. Hypothesis on the mechanism by which bloodborne IL-1 acts in the OVLT to produce fever. IL-1 would promote the formation of PGE_2 through the activation of neurons projecting to the adjoining hypothalamic region and of local reticuloendothelial cells. POM, medial preoptic nucleus; POME, median preoptic nucleus; CA, anterior commissure. (From Coceani, 1991.)

endotoxin and measured synthesis of what appeared to be IL-1 in their brains, possibly including the hypothalamus. Certainly, immunoreactive IL-1β has been found in the rat medial hypothalamus, periventricular region and fibres distributed to the hippocampus and olfactory tubercle (Lechan *et al.*, 1990) and it has been found in the human brain by Breder *et al.* (1988). IL-1-like activity has been shown to increase in the brain after brain injury (Nieto-Sampedro & Berman, 1987) and to be made in astrocytes. This should sound a warning about the use and interpretation of invasive techniques to recover brain cytokines, or products which they induce, because of the possible cellular damage produced by relatively large cannulae.

OVLT REGION

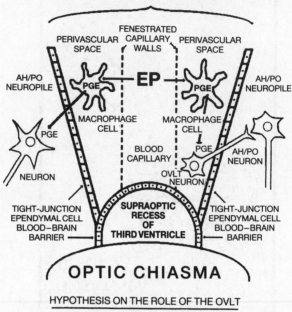

HYPOTHESIS ON THE ROLE OF THE OVLT
IN THE PATHOGENESIS OF FEVER

Fig. 5.6. An hypothesis on the role of the OVLT in the pathogenesis of fever. The diagram represents a coronal section of the AH/PO at the level of the supraoptic recess of the third ventricle, showing the OVLT, bounded on either side by the neuropile of the AH/PO. Endogenous pyrogen (EP) enters the perivascular spaces of the OVLT from the circulation through the fenestrated capillary walls and stimulates the mesenchymally derived cells (stellate-shaped cells) in the parenchyma to produce PGE. The PGE thus released into the OVLT is thought either to diffuse into the adjacent AH/PO region to cause fever (left-hand side), or to act upon neurons within the OVLT region to cause fever (right-hand side). (From Stitt, 1986.)

Morimoto *et al.* (1990) also postulated that in rats there are structural or functional differences between the blood–brain barrier of the extra-cerebral circulation and in the CNS as compared to the rabbit, and this makes it necessary to consider very carefully species differences in responses.

Studies which demonstrated a reduction in brainstem 5-HT content after giving intravenous bacterial pyrogen to rabbits suggested a possible role for this amine as a link in the fever pathway. A later suggestion was that there is a monoaminergic link from the OVLT to the hypothalamus involving 5-HT, and this has been explored by Shibata & Blatteis (in

Blatteis, 1992) in tissue slices from guinea-pigs. They found that neurons which were excited by 5-HT were also excited by TNF or IFN. However, in conscious guinea-pigs Blatteis (1992) reported that preoptic treatment with methysergide did not alter the expected fevers in response to endotoxin, and 5-HT dialysed into the AH/POA did not mimic fever (Quan *et al.*, 1991). So the 5-HT link looks unlikely. Blatteis *et al.* (1991, in Blatteis, 1992) found support for the possibility that substance-P containing neurons could be involved in the OVLT – preoptic area signal transduction. The full validation of this notion is not yet complete. So, the nature of the way in which the OVLT signals the thermoregulatory system in the hypothalamus is as yet an open question and a fruitful area for further research.

Actions of cytokines and prostaglandins in the hypothalamus

Responses of single neurons

Cabanac *et al.*, in 1968, studied the actions of temperature and intra-venous pyrogens on single units in the brain stem of urethane anaes-thetized rabbits. They identified warm sensitive and cold sensitive units the firing rates of which fell on 'bell shaped' curves. Intravenous typhoid vaccine inhibited warm sensitive units in 7 to 13 min and some cold sensitive units increased their firing rates in 17 to 21 min. The units tested in fever were hypothalamic. Witt & Wang (1968) identified temperature sensitive neurons in the AH/POA in the cat. Units which responded with an increased firing rate to hypothalamic heating had that increased firing rate reduced greatly when bacterial pyrogen was given into the internal carotid artery. Units which had had their firing rates depressed by pyrogen had them restored by intravenous administration of sodium salicylate. A similar result was obtained when both the pyrogen and salicylate were given into the carotid artery. These results added weight to the hypothesis that bacterial pyrogen, or the substances released by its actions could alter the behaviour of thermosensitive structures in the hypothalamus.

Eisenman (1969) also studied the effect of intravenous bacterial pyrogen on the thermosensitivity of neurons in the septum and the preoptic area in the urethane anaesthetized cat. Highly thermosensitive neurons ($Q_{10} > 2$), in the preoptic area had their thermosensitivities reduced by the pyrogen without any change in the basal firing rate at the usual core temperature of 38 °C. Warm sensitive units, possibly interneurons, had their thermosensitivities and firing rates reduced, and cold sensitive interneurons increased their firing rates in response to pyrogen. Thermally insensitive and neuron ($Q_{10} = 2$) firing rates did not alter.

That a depression of AH/POA thermosensitivity is caused by icv administration of killed *Salmonella typhosa* cells was demonstrated in the conscious rabbit by Eisenman (1974), in experiments in which he recorded the metabolic rate at 33 °C and 42 °C before and after pyrogen injections. Presumably the bacteria evoked release of cytokines. He also observed a depressed AH/POA thermosensitivity after intravenous pyrogen.

Thus far, the actions of pyrogens given iv, intra-arterially and icv have indicated appropriate alterations in the behaviour of thermosensitive neurons, if these are indeed part of the thermoregulatory mechanisms, for an increase in heat production and heat retention, and decreased heat loss in fever. However, the units which are responsible for the alteration in the apparent set point in fever are not known, but the action of pyrogens on what appear to be interneurons may be important in this regard.

What has been described so far in this section does, however, beg the question of what final fever mediator acts on thermosensitive hypothalamic structures, and how. There is some evidence that TNF-β can decrease the firing rate of warm sensitive neurons and that since this action is blocked with salicylate a PGE pathway is involved (Nakashima *et al.*, 1991). The putative mediator PGE$_2$ (or sometimes PGE$_1$), has been applied to hypothalamic neurons. The results are confusing. Schoener & Wang (1976) and Schoener (1980) report depression of warm units and excitation of cold firing units when 50 ng PGE$_1$ was topically applied to them, but at higher doses secondary reversal of these responses was observed. He also comments that others have used the discrete micro-iontophoresis application of prostaglandins with inconsistent results. Stitt (1981) reports the results of electrophoresis of PGE$_1$ onto warm and cold sensitive hypothalamic neurons and his findings are presented in Table 5.3. These results are not very convincing for the postulate that locally released, or diffused, prostaglandins are the fever mediator acting on thermosensitive neurons at the hypothalamic level. Hori *et al.* (1988) investigated the effect of iontophoretically applied IL-1 on the electrical activity of hypothalamic neurons. They found decreased activity in warm sensitive units, increased firing of cold sensitive units and no effect on thermally insensitive neurons. The responses of the

Table 5.3. *Effects of PGE$_1$ in anterior hypothalamus/preoptic units classified as warm-sensitive, cold-sensitive, or thermally insensitive*

Unit type	Total number tested	PGE$_1$- excited	PGE$_1$- depressed	No PGE$_1$ response
Warm-sensitive	63 (45.6)*	5 (8.0)	0 (0)	58 (92.0)
Cold-sensitive	10 (7.3)	1 (10.0)	0 (0)	9 (90.0)
Insensitive	65 (47.1)	6 (9.0)	0 (0)	59 (91.0)
Total units	138 (100)	12 (8.7)	0 (0)	126 (91.3)

*Numbers in parentheses are percentages.
(From Stitt, 1981.)

warm and cold sensitive neurons to IL-1 was blocked by phospholipase and cyclo-oxygenase inhibition suggesting that the IL-1 effects were prostaglandin mediated. Many interpretations are possible, the first being that local PGE released in the AH/POA is not the sole or ultimate thermoregulatory neuron mediator in fever; the second is that PGE$_2$ excites other cells, for example the postulated substance P-releasing neurons (Blatteis *et al.*, 1991 in Blatteis, 1992); a third is that a further and as yet unknown mediator is used. Xin & Blatteis (1992) showed that an anti-substance P compound blocked the effect of substance P on warm firing and insensitive preoptic slice neurons, and an IL-1β receptor antagonist blocked the effect of IL-1β on most warm and insensitive neurons but only blocked a small percentage of neurons treated with substance P. Indomethacin did not block the effects of substance P or IL-1β on warm or insensitive neurons. Out of these observations the authors suggested that substance P may be involved in the action of IL-1β on preoptic neurons and that it is unlikely to act by local induction of IL-1β or prostaglandins. As Eisenman (1982) has pointed out the iontophoresed PGE might not have reached the thermosensitive neurons whereas that given by intraventricular or micro-injection techniques would reach a larger population of neurons. Other possible explanations for the conflicting responses reported for the action of prostaglandins on thermosensitive neurons include the variety of anaesthetics used, and the chance that some thermosensitive neurons are not involved in thermoregulation and some are, and that many of the units studied could have belonged to one or other group. On the presently available evidence it seems clear that PGE_2 is an important intracerebral fever mediator, but that the responses of thermosensitive neurons are likely to be caused by a pathway which is PGE_2 stimulated and that the thermosensitive units may not be stimulated directly by the prostaglandins.

A peptide which acts in the pituitary gland is CRF, but it has multiple hypothalamic actions as well. One of these is on the thermogenic response to pyrogens (Rothwell, 1989). When injected into the brain it causes thermogenesis in BAT in rodents. Administration of PGE_2 and $PGF_{2\alpha}$ icv induced an increase in core temperature in rats which was accompanied by a rise in oxygen consumption (Rothwell, 1990). Large doses of CRF and these prostaglandins gave additive responses. A CRF receptor antagonist blocked the effects of $PGF_{2\alpha}$ but not of PGE_2 suggesting different mechanisms for the heat generation. It is also suggested that $PGF_{2\alpha}$ could be involved in IL-1β induced thermogenesis since it appears that the peptide may act via CRF (Rothwell, 1992). An antipyretic action of CRF administered into the CNS of rabbits has been reported (Bernadini *et al.*, 1984; Opp *et al.*, 1989). However, the difference in the amount and distribution of BAT in different species, with BAT contributing a large proportion of the heat excess in fever in some, makes direct comparison of responses to 'central' CRF dangerous. Another cytokine which can produce fever, accompanied by an increase in oxygen consumption, when injected into cerebral ventricles of rats is TNFα (Rothwell, 1988). She showed that these responses were principally dependent on the sympathetic outflow and that they were not dependent on CRF release.

A peripheral action of CRF was studied in rabbits (Milton *et al.*, 1993a). It was found that both CRF and PolyI:PolyC stimulated increases in PGE_2 and $PGE_{2\alpha}$ in the peripheral circulation of the conscious animal, and the response to the latter was blocked by the use of a CRF receptor antagonist or anti-CRF antibodies. So the fever modulating effect of peripheral CRF could be mediated by its effect on prostaglandin production.

Macrophage-type cells – astrocytes and microglia – are widely distributed in brain tissue and stimulation of these by injury or infection can release cytokines such as TNF and IL-1. They can be of great value in neuron protection and repair, but they can have deleterious effects, such as scar tissue formation, which can interfere with neuron sprouting.

The good/deleterious balance of the responses of these macrophages can be precarious (Piani *et al.*, 1994).

A role for hypothalamic monoamines?

Since the first proposal (Feldberg & Myers, 1963) that thermoregulation depended on the relative releases of noradrenaline and 5-HT in the hypothalamus, many studies have been made on numerous species to identify these amines with thermoregulatory function and their alteration in fever. The proposal was that thermoregulation depends on the relative rates of release from synapses in thermoregulatory pathways. Cooper (1965b) suggested that in the rabbit, in which noradrenaline infused into the hypothalamus had raised the body temperature, the action of pyrogens might be to augment the release of noradrenaline from hypothalamic thermoregulatory presynaptic junctions. In the cat, the hyperthermic amine 5-HT might subserve the same role. This comment was speculative. Cooper & Cranston (1966) reported that the monoamine oxidase inhibitor pargyline (N-benzyl-N-methyl-2-propynylamine) hydrochloride enhanced the febrile rise in temperature induced by leucocyte pyrogen. This compound causes accumulation of noradrenaline and potentiation of the action of tyramine (Goodman & Gilman, 1975). These observations would seem to suggest monoaminergic synapses in the fever neuronal pathway. Cooper *et al.* (1967) found that intraventricular reserpine in an amount which was shown to deplete the hypothalamus of noradrenaline (Cooper *et al.*, 1967) did not prevent fever in response to intravenous bacterial pyrogen in the rabbit suggesting that, in the rabbit, noradrenaline (the hyperthermic amine in this species) is not involved in synaptic transmission in the fever pathways. The evidence for this is suggestive but far from complete. A possible role for dopaminergic relays has yet to be determined and there is conflicting evidence for the participation of cholinergic pathways in fever (Cox & Lee, 1982). Cooper *et al.* (1976) found attenuation of PGE or leucocyte pyrogen induced fever by atropine given into a lateral cerebral ventricle in the rabbit, but the timing of the atropine administration was critical. Cranston (1979) pointed out that atropine given into the cerebral ventricles lowered core temperature and so the reduction in fever by intraventricular acetylcholine could just be the algebraic sum of the hypothermic action of the acetylcholine and the hyperthermic effect of the pyrogen, and not necessarily indicating a cholinergic pathway. Similar attenuation of fever by this muscarinic antagonist was reported for sheep (Bligh *et al.,* 1977) and for monkeys (Simpson *et al.,* 1977). Nicotinic antagonists have also been reported to attenuate fever in rabbits (Tangri *et al.,* 1974). There may be species differences for it seems that there is little evidence that cholinergic pathways play a role in fever in the rat. Teddy (1971) found that PCPA given into the brain, which depletes the brain of 5-HT, enhanced fever and noradrenaline depletion (caused by treatment with α-methylmetatyrosine), reduced fever in the rabbit. Alpha-methylparatyrosine, which is a tyrosine hydroxylase inhibitor, also reduced fever. Harvey & Milton (1974) found that PCPA reduced the response to intravenous and intraventricular pyrogen in conscious cats (a species in which 5-HT injected into the hypothalamus evokes hyperthermia), and the thermal response to intraventricular 5-HT and noradrenaline was unchanged. Direct injection of IL-1β into the anterior hypothalamus was found to increase the amounts of 5-HT, noradrenaline and dopamine into a micro-dialysis system in the same region in rats (Shintani *et al.,* 1993). They also found evidence that the augmented noradrenaline release was not dependent on prostaglandin or CRF involvement.

There is then evidence from the rather crude applications of monoamine altering substances into the brain and from monoamine recovery experiments that some part of the fever neuronal pathway uses monoamines as neurotransmitters but the evidence remains inconsistent and somewhat muddled. Many other functional pathways also appear to use monoamines as synaptic transmitters and we do not know for certain at this time which neurons, if any, in the dense tangle of hypothalamic fibres are solely devoted to thermoregulatory or to fever functions, or whether some fibres with many varicose terminals along their lengths may interconnect with neurons subserving several functions.

Alteration of the 'set point'

Since we do not know the actual neuronal mechanism or mechanisms that determine the body temperature set point it is difficult to postulate an action of pyrogens which would alter it. It is possible that the final fever mediator(s) could act on neurons outside the normal thermoregulatory pathways but which impinge on the efferent mechanisms in such a way that the heat production and conservation pathways are stimulated and the crossed-over heat loss pathways inhibited. This could occur until the core temperature is raised to a limit determined by the concentration of fever mediator at the efferent system centre at which point the normally functioning thermodetection and its efferent outflow could again induce thermoregulatory responses at the higher temperature level. That the thermoregulatory system can function quantitatively and in the normal manner at a higher than usual temperature in fever has been demonstrated in the human. Macpherson (1959) showed that a subject exercising in a hot room during a bout of influenzal fever had patterns of change in core temperature at the febrile level during exercise which exactly paralleled those seen when afebrile (Fig. 1.1), and the sweat rate responses to exercise were identical. Cooper *et al.* (1964c) were able to demonstrate that the hand blood-flow responses to body core warming were exactly the same at the plateau of fever induced by iv pyrogen as they were in the same subjects tested when afebrile (see Chapter 1). Some have implicated an alteration in the balance of Na^+ to Ca^{++} ions in the posterior hypothalamus with a shift to an excess of Na^+ ions as a cause of the raised set point in fever (Myers & Tytell, 1972, and reviewed by Myers, 1982) and certainly ion fluxes which are in the right direction have been reported by these authors to occur in fever. From a study in which high Ca^{++} containing artificial csf was infused into monkey cerebral ventricles at widely differing environmental temperatures Gisolfi *et al.* (1983) could not find evidence for a set point function for Ca^{++}. It failed to induce the physiological responses consistent with changes in temperature set point at the differing environmental temperatures. The possibility that the ion fluxes may not be the primary determinants of temperature set point but that they may modulate synaptic events which are in the actual set point network has been suggested; and interpretation of the ion flux *vis à vis* the synaptic responses to altered levels of the ions is difficult to correlate (Cranston, 1979).

The efferent systems

General comments

The main functions which are modified in fever include the constriction of skin blood vessels, shivering and non-shivering heat production augmentation, inhibition of sweating, behavioural to bring about heat conservation, and the modification of peripheral plasma metallic ions and immune products. Those functions which depend on the outflow of the sympathetic nervous system such as the enhancing of heat production in BAT and peripheral vasomotor responses depend on innervation by sympathetic fibres the cell bodies of which are located in the paravertebral sympathetic ganglia. Their preganglionic fibres have their cells of origin in the intermediolateral cell columns of the spinal cord. Some visceral functions which are involved in fever and are under sympathetic nervous control may also have postganglionic fibres originating in the mesenteric, coeliac and other intra-abdominal ganglia. Their preganglionic connections also have cell bodies in the intermediolateral columns of the spinal cord.

A general scheme of connections of the hypothalamus is shown in Fig 5.7 which is taken from Palkovits & Záborszky (1979) but the pathways from the thermoregulatory regions of the septum, the hypothalamus and brainstem to the intermediolateral columns or the motor outflow from the spinal cord are not well defined as yet. HRP injected into the spinal cord in rats, cats and the monkey (*Macaca fasciculus*) was found by Saper *et al*. (1976b) to be transported, mostly ipsilaterally, from T_7–T_{12} to the PVN and also to the dorsolateral hypothalamus, the dorsal and dorsomedial hypothalamic areas, the posterior hypothalamus dorsal to the mamillary body and the central grey. There is an anatomical pathway from the paraventricular nucleus to the intermediolateral column of the spinal cord but its function is not known. Using a different anterogradely transported marker, *Phaseolus vulgaris* leuco-agglutinin, Luiten *et al*. (1985) investigated efferent neurons having their cells of origin in the paraventricular nucleus. One marked tract went to the periventricular grey area and another to the ventral reticular formation. Fibres of both bundles coursed through the pons and medulla, and some terminated in the nucleus of the tractus solitarius and some in the area postrema, and at the spinal-level fibres were distributed over the length of the spinal cord down to the lumbar region with connections to the intermediolateral columns. Again the precise visceral functions of these fibres cannot be stated. Connections from the PVN to the sympathetic preganglionic neurons in the upper part of the thoracic region of the rat spinal cord were also demonstrated by Hosoya *et al*. (1991). There are said to be substance P-containing neurons, and met-enkephalin containing neurons, connecting the medial preoptic area to the PVN. Electrophysiological techniques were used by Yamashita *et al*. (1984), to demonstrate monosynaptic connections between the PVN and the intermediolateral columns of the thoracic region of the spinal cord in cats, but the autonomic functions which they subserve are

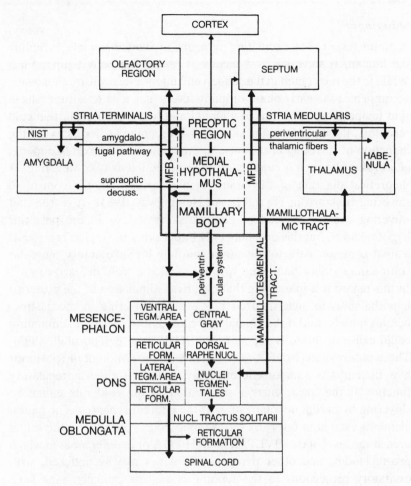

Fig. 5.7. Summary of efferent connections of the hypothalamus. (From Palkovits & Záborszky, 1979.)

not known. Again, Pittman *et al.* (1981), using electrophysiological methods, showed the existence of connections between the rat PVN and the amygdala, the lateral septum, the median eminence and the peri-aqueductal grey. So while many anatomical connections have been demonstrated, the correlations of these with a function have been far less impressive. The efferent connections of the hypothalamus are many and to diverse parts of the CNS and one version of these is shown in Fig. 5.7 taken from Palkovits & Záborszky (1979).

Shivering

A major response to circulating pyrogens in many mammals, including the human, is shivering as a means of raising the body temperature. While in the intact human the sudden and intense vasoconstriction which accompanies the early phase of many fevers may lead to abrupt falls in skin temperatures and thus to a large input to the brain from skin cold receptors, the input from the skin does not seem to be necessary for the induction of shivering in response to intravenous endotoxin (Cooper *et al.*, 1964a) although it could contribute to the intensity of shivering. A theoretical diagram of the brain regions involved in the control of shivering is shown in Fig 5.8 (from Hemingway, 1963). It is true that shivering can be reduced or eliminated by lesions in the posterior hypothalamus, but this probably only implies that the region represents a final common path to the motor outflow for involuntary muscular contractions rather than what was once called a 'cold defence centre'. In this regard it is interesting that electrical stimulation of the posterior hypothalamus in anaesthetized rats evoked shivering in the gastrocnemius muscle, and if the animal was cooled, lower current stimulation could cause or intensify the shivering (Halvorson & Thornhill, 1993). These observations would be consistent with the notion of the posterior hypothalamus as a major efferent relay station for a thermoregulatory function if the lower current stimulation in the cold rats enhanced shivering by partial depolarization at the efferent synapses. The neural elements excited in fever, by for example PGE_2, could be in the septal area at the level of the OVLT, in the AH/POA or in other areas in which prostaglandins and other pyrogenic cytokines may be induced, with excitatory projections to the septum as well as caudally. Any such proposed pathways lack functional anatomical demonstration and are speculative.

Non-shivering thermogenesis – BAT

Interesting studies by Imai-Matsumura & Nakayama (1987) examined the BAT thermogenesis during preoptic cooling in the rat following bilateral micro-injections of local anaesthetic into parts of the hypothalamus. Preoptic cooling increased both BAT and colonic temperatures. Lidocaine injected into the ventromedial hypothalamus reduced and injected into the anterior hypothalamus increased BAT temperature. The injection of lidocaine into the lateral hypothalamus was without effect as were saline control injections. The authors

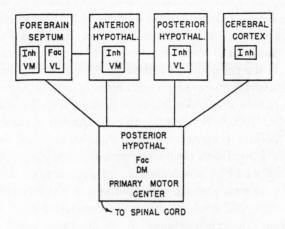

Fig. 5.8. Nervous control of shivering with primary motor centre in rostral (posterior) hypothalamus and subsidiary (secondary) control centres elsewhere. Inh, inhibitory; Fac, facilitatory; V, ventral; M, medial; D, dorsal; L, lateral. (From Hemingway, 1963.)

proposed that the pathway from the preoptic area to BAT traverses the medial part of the hypothalamus and that the ventromedial hypothalamus facilitates and the anterior hypothalamus inhibits BAT thermogenesis. Presumably this pathway could be used in the rat for increasing BAT thermogenesis in response to pyrogens. Evidence has been found to suggest that the NTS is an important relay in the outflow of the sympathetic system to BAT and is used in BAT thermogenesis in fever caused by intraventricular PGE_1 (Fyda *et al.*, 1991). These authors made bilateral electrolytic lesions in the NTS and the lesions attenuated the rise normally occurring in metabolic rate, core temperature and BAT temperature in response to the prostaglandin. The efferent pathway to BAT includes the intermediolateral columns of the spinal cord, the preganglionic sympathetic fibres which have their cell bodies there and the postganglionic β-adrenergic fibres which innervate the BAT.

Vasomotor responses, pilomotor changes and sweating

Intense vasoconstriction accompanies the rising phase of fever in the human and in many other mammals. In the *extremities* vasoconstriction is brought about by an increase in impulse traffic along the α-adrenergic post-ganglionic fibres to the skin blood vessels. Their pre-ganglionic connections have their cell bodies in the intermediolateral columns of the spinal cord. While anatomically determined pathways from the OVLT and AH/POA to the intermediolateral columns can be demonstrated, the possibility that those pathways are the ones used in pyrogen induced vasomotor responses cannot at present be proven. The vasoconstriction in other skin areas is presumed to be due both to *inhibition of vasodilator* fibres and perhaps excitation of vasoconstrictor neurons with little known about their relative function in pyrogen induced fever. Sympathetic cholinergic post-ganglionic neurons to sweat glands are inhibited by a process which starts in the brain with nothing known of its pathway through the brainstem to the intermediolateral columns of the spinal cord. Likewise the cholinergic pathways to the arrectores pili, the pre-ganglionic fibres of which come from the intermediolateral columns of the spinal cord, have higher control routes which are virtually unknown.

Fever in animals in which thermoregulation is impaired by anaesthesia

Siren (1982) reported fever in rats that were anaesthetized with urethane and which were given PGE_2 into their lateral ventricles. Previously, experiments were done to test the effects of anaesthesia on fever produced by iv endotoxin or icv PGE_2 (Dashwood & Feldberg, 1977). Pentobarbitone sodium anaesthetized cats were able to get fever in response to endotoxin but the response was diminished, and chloralose blocked the fever. PGE_2 was able to induce fever in chloralose anaesthetized as well as pentobarbitone sodium anaesthetized cats but again the response was reduced. A detailed study of the thermoregulatory control and the ability to develop fever was made using urethane anaesthetized rats (Malkinson *et al.*, 1988). The anaesthetic, given so as to maintain a stage III, plane I level of anaesthesia, abolished the ability of the animals to regulate their body temperatures. Exposed to an ambient temperature of 32 °C the rats' temperatures rose abruptly and continued to rise until they were removed from the heat, and at 9 °C ambient temperature the animals' core temperatures fell precipitously. The core temperatures also fell at 22 °C ambient but at this temperature by placing the animal on a heating pad its core temperature could be held reasonably steady by manually adjusting the electric current flowing through the pad and, at equilibrium, leaving it at the equilibrium setting. At lower ambient temperatures there was usually a small fall in the animal's core temperature during the resting control period. However, administration of PGE_1 into a lateral cerebral ventricle or into the AH/POA resulted in the characteristic fever reaction with a rise in core temperature even when the resting core temperature was as low as 33 °C or as high as 39 °C. IL-1 given into a lateral cerebral ventricle also produced fever in the urethane anaesthetized rat. The rises in core temperature were greatest when the pyrogen was given at a resting core temperature of about 32–34 °C and least when the core temperature was just over 39 °C. The temperature responses of rats under urethane anaesthesia to PGE_1 at various pre-administration temperatures are shown in Fig. 5.9. So, the effector mechanisms for raising the core temperature in response to pyrogen challenge are clearly still available in the urethane anaesthetized rat. It is known (Witt & Wang, 1968; Eisenman, 1969; Gottschlich *et al.*, 1984) that hypothalamic thermosensitive neurons can function under anaesthesia and consequently if we can assume that these sensors are part of the normal thermoregulatory apparatus the afferent information necessary for thermoregulation functions under the anaesthesia. The fact that peripheral vasoconstriction and shivering was observed in the pyrogen treated anaesthetized rats is consistent not only with relatively intact efferent systems, assuming the reported action of pyrogenic cytokines on thermosensitive units to be relevant, but also with the probability of relative intactness of the afferent thermal information systems. The pyrogens, or some substance(s) in the intracerebral response cascade, could act directly on the efferent pathways to stimulate heat production and heat retention but bypassing the central controller. The pyrogenic substance could possibly act at a locus outside the normal thermoregulatory pathway which could secondarily drive the efferent systems. It could act on the midbrain arousal system to raise the level of depolarization of the efferent neuron pools, but there was no evidence for other aspects of general arousal (indeed IL-1 may induce somnolence), or it is possible that the pyrogens could act on links between the thermodetectors and the central controller which are depressed by the anaesthetic. The interesting part of these observations is the dissociation of thermoregulatory control from the process of fever, and further investigation of this could shed new light on both processes.

It is always good to see the application of new techniques to the elucidation of difficult physiological problems. One such – the expression of the nuclear proto-oncogene c-fos – which can be studied by immunostaining for c-fos protein, can often detect activation of neuronal cell bodies (Dragunow & Faull, 1989). This has now been used by

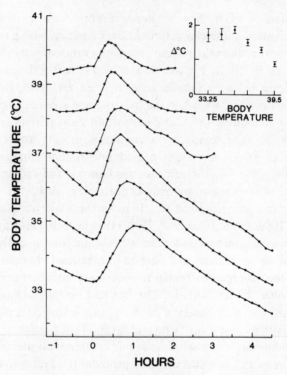

Fig. 5.9. Colonic temperature responses to icv PGE, in urethane anaesthetized rats, starting at different body temperatures. Inset: the maximum rise in core temperature plotted against resting temperature. (From Malkinson *et al.*, 1988.)

Oladehin *et al.* (1994), to study the regions of the brain which become active in response to intravenous endotoxin with careful controls to reduce the effect of stress on the interpretation of the data. It was clear that increased immunostaining for c-fos protein occurred in the septum in response to the endotoxin, the preoptic area, other hypothalamic regions, the thalamus, the bed nucleus of the stria terminalis and to a lesser but very significant extent in the amygdala and the NTS. Thus, not only was there activity in the hypothalamic thermoregulatory regions, but also in regions thought to be associated with endogenous antipyresis, e.g., the BST and the amygdala. The NTS is known as a region involved in the activation of BAT, a potent source of heat production during fever in the rat. Interestingly, the regions adjacent to the OVLT, the subfornical organ and the area postrema were also labelled though the actual organs were not. Another investigation (Rivest *et al.*, 1992) to study other neuroendocrine functions found that IL-1β given to castrated male rats iv did not alter c-fos protein expression in the PVN or arcuate nucleus, however, when given icv, c-fos expression in the PVN and arcuate nucleus was augmented. It is interesting that the PVN and the arcuate nucleus are loci of origins of neurons containing two endogenous antipyretics, but the apparent activation of presynaptic terminals only on icv pyrogen and not on iv pyrogen administration is curious. One must also remember that the animals used were castrated and thus the pattern of AVP neuron content was likely to be abnormal. Clearly the exact conditions under which such studies are made needs very careful delineation and control. Other studies will be done with this technique and they will provide useful information for the design of electrophysiological studies in fever. If the c-fos expression can be induced in the urethane anaesthetized rat this will provide another means of dissociating stress responses from the effects of pyrogenic cytokines and other fever mediators.

6

The role of the cerebral cortex, the limbic system, peripheral nervous system and spinal cord and induced changes in intracranial pressure

The cerebral cortex and limbic system

Functional roles for parts of the cerebral cortex in the control of autonomic nervous system activity have been suspected and partially demonstrated for several decades. Fulton (1949) describes autonomic representation in the pre-central motor cortex. Newman & Wolstencroft (1960) found that heating the blood flowing in the carotid arteries to about 41 °C caused a fall in arterial blood pressure, presumably associated with peripheral vasodilatation, and that stimulation of the posterior orbital cortex prevented the fall in blood pressure. Ström (1950) reported that electrical stimulation of the frontal cortex and also the hypothalamus elicited peripheral vasoconstriction in dogs, cats and rabbits, but frontal decortication did not abolish the vasoconstriction consequent on hypothalamic stimulation implying that the hypothalamically induced vasoconstriction did not depend on a cortical pathway. Eliasson & Ström (1950) located the cortical vasoconstrictor region to a region close to the cruciate sulcus and in the white matter of the frontal lobe. A full discussion of the association of various cortical areas with autonomic function has been published by Cechetto & Saper (1990). Dogs which are decorticated have impaired body temperature regulation in both hot and cold environments (Pinkston et al., 1934; Delgado & Livingstone, 1948). A method for functional decortication is the induction of CSD by flooding an area of the cerebral cortex with high molarity K^+ solution. This has been shown to alter thermoregulatory functions in rats (Shibata et al., 1983, 1984, 1985). Monda et al. (1992) were able to demonstrate that CSD blocked the nervous activation of interscapular BAT during PGE_1 induced fever. The effect of CSD on fever induced by icv administration of PGE_1 and also to intravenous endotoxin was studied, in conscious male rats, by Monda & Pittman (1993). They found that CSD profoundly reduced both types of fever, particularly in the initial rapid phase. In their experiments, CSD did not alter body temperature in afebrile animals, an observation which agrees with the work of De Luca *et al.* (1987). This work was extended by Komáromi *et al.* (1994). They found that CSD induced in rats reduced the fever induced by icv PGE_1 in doses 30 and 60 ng in the conscious rat and 90 ng in the urethane anaesthetized rat. The reduction in body temperature rise was accompanied by a marked reduction in O_2 uptake in the anaesthetized animals. CSD was without effect on core temperature in animals not having fever induced. These experiments indicate a possible role for the cerebral cortex in fever. There was good reason to suspect that the reduction in fever was not due to sudden depolarization of cortico-septal connections leading to a large septal release of AVP, a putative endogenous antipyretic, since the fever reduction has been observed in castrated rats in which the AVP stores are depleted (Komáromi *et al.* 1994). The pathways involved in the cortical interaction with fever processes are not known, neither is it known whether CSD alters other aspects of the acute phase reaction. The sensory cortex would also be expected to play a role in behavioural responses to the conscious awareness of severe cold sensation, headache and occasional photophobia that accompany many abrupt severe fevers.

The complex connections between the hypothalamic nuclei and the amygdala, the septal areas and the bed nucleus of the stria terminalis all of which are interconnected have been discussed in Chapter 5. That these areas could be involved in both autonomic and behavioural febrile responses is both possible and likely, and their involvement in endogenous antipyresis is described in Chapter 7.

The peripheral nerves and spinal cord

The peripheral nervous system provides afferent information related to the skin temperature and also sensory information which can lead to unpleasant aching in muscles and joints in fever. In some species (including human infants) the efferent nerves provide commands to the muscles to initiate and maintain shivering, to turn on heat production in BAT, to constrict skin blood vessels and to bring about the behavioural responses used in fever. In addition, during the defervescence they are used to cause peripheral vasodilatation, sweating and heat losing behavioural responses.

There is evidence that peripherally developed pyrogens do not act on

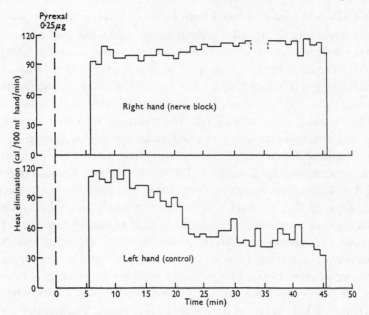

Fig. 6.1. Heat elimination measured simultaneously from both hands after intravenous pyrogen. Right hand = complete nerve block; left hand = control. (From Bryce-Smith *et al.*, 1959.)

peripheral nerves, on vascular smooth muscle or on elements in the isolated spinal cord. Bryce-Smith *et al.* (1959) completely blocked the nerves to the right hand of a human subject with lignocaine, and then measured the heat elimination from both hands by calorimetry (for this method see Greenfield, 1960a,b). The room was so warm that the initial heat eliminations from the two hands were similar. The heat elimination is a good measure of the blood flow averaged over one minute. Six minutes after the start of blood flow recordings began, the subject received an intravenous injection of 50 ml of his own blood which had been incubated for 2.5 hours after being mixed with 0.3 μg of *Salmonella abortus equi* endotoxin. The blood flow in the control hand fell markedly (Fig. 6.1) at a time when the fever commenced and was rising. The blood flow in the nerve-blocked hand did not alter significantly.

Thus the vasoconstriction which accompanies fever, and which is in part responsible for the increase in body temperature, is not due to a direct action of the injected endogenous pyrogen on the peripheral sympathetic nerve terminals on the blood vessels, or on the vascular smooth muscle.

A young man who had a physiologically complete lesion of his spinal cord at C6–C7 received an intravenous injection of 50 ml of his own blood which had been incubated with the endotoxin from *S. abortus equi* (0.05 μg) and his core temperatures as well as his hand and finger blood flows were measured. Surface and subcutaneous temperatures were measured on his chest. Deltoid muscle electromyograph recordings were also made (Cooper *et al.*, 1964a). There was no consequent vasoconstriction in the finger or hand. Slight increases in core temperature (0.1 °C in one experiment and 0.3–0.5 °C in a second) were noted. The trunk skin temperatures remained warm and his face remained flushed. He did not experience headache. There was marked shivering in the muscles innervated from above the lesion but none in the rest of the musculature. Again, since the lesion was above the outflow of sympathetic fibres from the cord, the absence of vasoconstriction indicates no action of the peripheral pyrogen mediator(s) on the sympathetic ganglia, the pre- or post-ganglionic fibres or on the intermedio-lateral columns in the isolated cord. The lack of shivering in the muscles innervated from below the lesion suggests no muscle contracting action of the pyrogens on anterior horn cells or elsewhere in the isolated cord. The lack of action of the pyrogens on the isolated cord does not rule out possible actions, particularly on afferent systems in the intact spinal cord. Action of pyrogens on afferent fibres entering the isolated cord, if it occurs, does not seem to elicit vasomotor or muscular responses. The absence of headache, which almost always occurs in subjects with no neurological deficits, is interesting. It could be linked to the absence of peripheral vasoconstriction and the consequent rise in intracranial pressure, which is normally seen in fever (Malkinson *et al.*, 1985).

In order to test whether the entry of some afferent thermal information involved in reflex vasodilatation, or the efferent arc of the reflex was suppressed during pyrogen fever, a simple experiment was performed (Bryce-Smith *et al.*, 1959). The blood flow was measured by venous occlusion plethysmography in both hands. After making baseline observations for 20 min either saline or endotoxin was injected intravenously. At the onset of the pyrogen-induced fever there was marked vasoconstriction in both hands. At this time the water surrounding the right hand was raised to 40 °C+, while that surrounding the left hand remained at 32 °C. The resting blood flow in the right hand, which had been close to zero in water at 32 °C, increased to a measurable level and the application of radiant heat to the trunk elicited reflex vasodilatation in that hand but not in the hand immersed in water at 32 °C (Fig. 6.2).

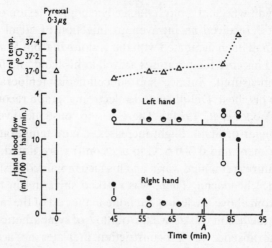

Fig. 6.2. Blood flows in right and left hands after intravenous Pyrexal. Both hands were initially in water at 32 °C. At A the water temperature in the right plethysmograph was raised to 42 °C. Radiant heat to trunk at arrow. (From Bryce-Smith *et al.*, 1959.)

Thus it appeared that the entire reflex vasodilatation pathway, which involves afferents which travel with the sympathetic nerves to the spinal cord and which appear to ascend at least to the posterior hypothalamus and probably beyond, were fully functional during the vasoconstriction phase of fever. The reflex response which was masked by the large efferent sympathetic vasoconstrictor tone was revealed by removing the effect of the increased sympathetic tone by local hand warming. One could postulate that the efferent sympathetic tone might be related to hand blood flow on a sigmoid curve (Fig. 6.3) with a negative slope and that in the rising phase of fever the sympathetic tone is high and far to the right. Until local warming directly relaxes the vascular smooth muscle and shifts the curve to the right to produce a significant resting blood-flow, the radiant heat-induced reduction in impulses to the vessels would not result in vasodilatation. This is hypothetical but possibly worth investigating as new methods for assessing the impulse traffic in peripheral sympathetic nerves become available. It is not known whether a similar unmasking of a peripheral vasodilatation would occur in response to raising the temperature of the 'hypothalamic' warm receptors during the vasoconstriction phase of fever.

During the rising phase of body temperature in fever, sweating is inhibited (Bannister, 1960; Table 6.1). Presumably there is cessation of the sympathetic impulses to the sweat glands although there are no

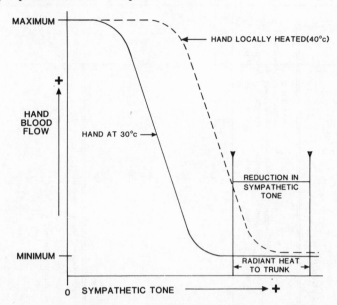

Fig. 6.3. A theoretical plot of hand blood-flow against tone in the sympathetic nerves to hand blood-vessels during fever, and the responses of these variables to radiant heat applied to the trunk. The solid line is with the hand in water at 30 °C and the dotted line is with the hand at 40 °C.

reported measurements of these. At the start of the falling phase of body temperature shivering stops, there is vasodilatation in the skin and sweating, often profuse, occurs. It is said that when the action of the endogenous mediators of fever ceases the 'set point' for body tempera-ture falls and the heat loss mechanisms are invoked with suppression of heat production, particularly shivering. The role of the peripheral nerves in the responses of defervescence of fever appears to be limited to carrying the altered impulse traffic to the peripheral effector organs.

During many febrile episodes the patient suffers aching pains in the muscles and sometimes the joints, and the skin may seem tender to touch. There is at present no clear evidence as to whether these sensory anomalies derive from unusual impulse traffic in the afferent nerves from skin or deeper tissues, or whether there is modification of the normal afferent traffic within some part of the CNS. This could be a fruitful future area of research.

One well-established accompaniment of fever induced by bacterial pyrogens is renal vasodilatation (Chassis *et al.*, 1938) and this has been reported to be unaffected by renal sympathectomy (Goldring *et al.*,

Table 6.1. *Effect of intravenous bacterial pyrogen on body temperature and sweating*

Experiment number	Days after first experiment	Subject	Control	Dose of pyrogen (μg)	Change of body temperature 2 hours after pyrogen (°F)*	Latency of initial change of oral temperature (minutes)	Decline of sweating†	Complete cessation of sweating	Latency of cessation (minutes)	Activation by intracutaneous methacholine chloride (where given)	Duration of cessation of sweating (minutes)
1	0	R.B.	J.M.	i 0.1	0.2	95	+	0		:	
				ii 0.2	2.9	60	+	+	60	+	50
2	10	R.B.	J.M.	0.25	0.4	80	+	+	80	+	10
3	89	R.B.	W.L.	0.30	1.2	80	0	0		:	
4	92	R.B.	G.N.	i 0.15	0	80	+	+	55	+	60
				ii 0.25	3.4	55	:	:		:	
5‡	112	R.B.	J.M.	i 0.15	0.2	105	+	+	90	+	60
				ii 0.25	4.0	60	+	+	90	:	7
6	124	R.B.	G.N.	0.45	1.0	90	+	+	90	:	15
7	18	J.M.	R.B.	0.2	0.1	95	:	:		:	
8	40	J.M.	R.B.	0.3	0.1	100	:	:		:	
9	47	W.L.	R.B.	0.2	0.5	85	+	0	85	+	45
10	43	W.L.	R.B.	i 0.1	0.7	85	+	+	105	+	18
				ii 0.2	2.1	105	+	+		+	
11	130	I.McC.	R.B.	0.15	0		+	+		+	

*Difference between body-temperature change in test subject and control, measured by subtraction of the difference between the mean temperature $\frac{(\text{oral} + \text{rectal})}{2}$ of subject and control at the time of the pyrogen injection from the difference two hours after the injection.

†Decline defined as a sweat loss (recorded as weight loss) two hours after the pyrogen injection less than 60% of the peak sweat loss.

‡Mean effective environmental temperature 73°F.

(From Bannister, 1960.)

1941). Cranston *et al.* (1959) showed that the increase in effective renal plasma flow resulting from pyrogens in the dog, occurred when the pyrogen was administered intrathecally and was not an effect of circulating bacterial pyrogen. The vasodilatation was investigated in a dog in which one kidney was removed and in which the other kidney was auto-transplanted into the pelvis. This made sure that the renal nerves were all severed (Cooper *et al.*, 1960). In this animal, intrathecal bacterial pyrogen caused fever accompanied by renal vasodilatation. In the same animal it was shown that the renal vasodilatation was not a consequence of the rise in body temperature, which if anything reduced the effective renal plasma flow and the total effective renal blood flow. The renal vasodilatation was due to an action of pyrogen within the CNS, was independent of the integrity of the nerves to the kidney and was clearly humorally mediated. The nature of the circulating renal vasodilatory substance is still not known. It is possible that it could act on an intra-renal nerve plexus but this waits to be determined. There is also an increase in hepatic blood flow in endotoxin-induced fever (Bradley & Conan, 1947), but the role, if any, of the nervous system in this vasodilatation is not known.

An intriguing result of denervation of the carotid bifurcation region on endotoxin-induced fever has been reported (Dascalu *et al.*, 1989). The experiments were performed on young lambs. Carotid (presumably either carotid sinus, carotid body or both) denervation suppressed fever in lambs given intravenous *S. abortus equi* purified endotoxin. The rise in O_2 uptake which accompanied fever in the control animals was significantly less in the denervated ones. The neural mechanism of this effect is not known though it is tempting to consider a connection between the carotid sinus input and the output to BAT from the nucleus solitarius, but such thoughts are only speculative.

ICP changes in fever

The separation of changes in ICP, in clinical situations, due to the effects of the fever process from those caused by other pathological changes such as in meningitis is difficult. It is possible to monitor continuously both icv and subarachnoid pressures during experimentally induced fever in conscious and anaesthetized animals. Malkinson *et al.* (1985) measured the pressure in a lateral cerebral ventricle in conscious cats and rabbits, and subarachnoid pressure in the conscious rabbit before and after iv administration of endotoxin (the lipopolysaccharide from

Table 6.2. *Maximum changes in body temperature (°C) and ICP or LCVP (mm saline) with administration of control artificial cerebrospinal fluid (aCSF) or control intravenous saline and doses of two pyrogenic agents*

A. Effect of PEG_1 fever upon ICP and LCVP in the urethane anaesthetized rat

PGE_1 into the LCV

	Temperature		ICP		
aCSF	0.05 (0.07)		−2.10	(3.60)	
100 ng	0.70 (0.17)	<0.01	21.90	(2.60)	<0.001
400 ng	1.68 (0.07)	<0.001	41.20	(5.10)	<0.001
	Temperature		LCVP		
aCSF	0.01 (0.14)		3.86	(3.58)	
100 ng	0.77 (0.09)	<0.001	30.89	(5.87)	<0.01
400 ng	1.56 (0.12)	<0.001	51.91	(4.54)	<0.001

PGE_1 into the AH/POA

	Temperature		ICP		
aCSF	−0.03 (0.09)		3.15	(3.36)	
10 ng	0.76 (0.15)	<0.01	13.64	(3.75)	<0.01
40 ng	1.33 (0.18)	<0.01	37.92	(6.04)	<0.001
	Temperature		LCVP		
aCSF	−0.09 (0.12)		−4.39	(3.63)	
10 ng	0.91 (0.11)	<0.001	16.70	(1.62)	<0.001
40 ng	1.28 (0.13)	<0.001	42.67	(5.97)	<0.001

B. Effect of PGE_1 fever upon LCVP in the conscious rat

PGE_1 into the LCV

	Temperature		LCVP		
aCSF	−0.17 (0.15)		2.10	(10.99)	
100 ng	1.10 (0.18)	<0.001	47.10	(11.16)	<0.05
800 ng	2.05 (0.11)	<0.001	91.70	(12.07)	<0.001

C. Effect of intravenous bacterial endotoxin fever upon ICP and LCVP in the conscious rabbit

	Temperature		ICP		
Saline	0.25 (0.07)		3.20	(1.78)	
0.025 µg/kg	1.84 (0.11)	<0.05	14.30	(3.01)	<0.05
	Temperature		LCVP		
Saline	0.07 (0.08)		−9.31	(8.67)	
0.0075 µg/kg	1.02 (0.12)	<0.05	19.86	(4.77)	<0.05

D. Effect of intravenous bacterial endotoxin fever upon LCVP in the conscious cat

	Temperature		LCVP		
Saline	0.24 (0.09)		−4.33	(11.22)	
0.02 µg/kg	1.56 (0.13)	<0.05	36.83	(4.11)	<0.05

Values represent the mean ± standard error of the mean from groups of ten rats or groups of six rabbits or cats. Significance from control experiments utilized single factor Analysis of Variance.
(From Malkinson *et al.*, 1993.)

Salmonella abortus equi). They found that both pressures in the rabbit and the ventricular pressure in the cat rose significantly during the rising temperature (chill) phase of fever. The ventricular and subarachnoid pulses increased in amplitude at the same time. Simultaneously there were increases in heart rate, arterial blood pressure and central venous pressure in the unanaesthetized rabbits, as well as a fall in ear skin temperature and respiratory rate. The arterial blood P_aCO_2 fell during the chill and flush phases of fever. The fall in arterial blood P_aCO_2 at a time when oxygen consumption is greatly raised must imply, despite the fall in respiratory rate, a considerable increase in pulmonary alveolar ventilation even accounting for any fall in respiratory quotient. The ventricular pressure, arterial pressure and venous pressures fell during the flush phase, and the ear skin temperature and respiratory rate rose at this time. A further study using urethane anaesthetized rats confirmed and extended the above findings (Malkinson *et al.*, 1988) on ICP, heart rate, blood pressure and P_aCO_2 during fever induced by PGE_1 injected into the lateral cerebral ventricle or the AH/POA, but in this preparation the respiratory rate rose. Control injections ruled out a significant effect of the volume of injected fluid on the ICP. A summary of the changes in intracranial and lateral cerebral ventricular pressures in rats, cats and rabbits using two pyrogenic agents is given in Table 6.2, taken from Malkinson *et al.* (1993). The rise in ICP during the chill, or rising temperature phase of temperature, could in part be related to the massive peripheral vasoconstriction with consequent increases in central venous pressure and arterial blood pressure, both of which could be exacerbated by vigorous shivering. The change in ICP evoked by pyrogens could play a part in the headache usually experienced in the chill phase of abrupt fevers. The observations related earlier in this chapter of the lack of headache in the patient with a high spinal cord lesion during pyrogen-induced 'fever' would be consistent with the postulate of a role for the peripheral vasoconstriction in the causation of the headache.

7
Antipyresis

Definition of antipyresis

As described in Chapter 1, in true fever the thermoregulatory system behaves as though there is a body temperature set point which is raised as part of the febrile process. Thus, in the plateau phase of fever raising or lowering the body core temperature evokes defence responses similar to those evoked at the 'normal' body temperature. In the febrile condition, as defined thus, administration of some drugs lowers the apparent set point for body temperature regulation and consequently reduces the body temperature. In other conditions, e.g., artificial body heating, exposure to high environmental heat stress, and more controversially during exercise, the body core temperature is raised but the apparent body temperature set point is not. Drugs that act to reduce true febrile temperature and which do not have an effect on normal body temperature or on the cooling rate of artificially, but not pathologically raised core temperature, are known as antipyretics. Some drugs are capable of reducing the core temperature without resetting the apparent set point, e.g., substances which under any circumstances will induce massive peripheral vasodilatation or profuse sweating may act to reduce core temperature in fever or under afebrile conditions. Amidopyrine, which has been used as an antipyretic, does cause a fall in core temperature in the afebrile rabbit, in a dose-dependent manner, with the maximum fall in core temperature in response to 100 mg intravenously of 0.35 °C (Grundmann, 1969). Others, such as barbiturates, anaesthetics and phenothiazines may lower body temperature by disrupting the brain thermoregulatory systems. These are not truly antipyretics. The definition given above does not consider the mechanisms of action of antipyretics and indeed an antipyretic may have a primary action on the temperature set point or it may induce indirect reduction

100

of the set point by, for example, release of an endogenous material which is the ultimate mediator of the antipyretic action. There are therefore some grey areas in the definition of an antipyretic substance.

Antipyretic drugs

Historical notes

Agents which reduce febrile body temperature have been known since ancient times. Both Hippocrates and Galen were aware of the temperature-lowering effects of extracts of the willow (*Salix alba*) (Gross & Greenberg, 1948). The ability of extracts of the bark of the cinchona plant (*Cinchona succiruba*) to 'cure' malaria and bring down the body temperature in that disease was known early in the 1600s in Peru where the plant grows. The name of the plant is said to derive from an apocryphal story – the Spanish countess of Cinchón introduced the plant to Spain after her husband, the viceroy of Peru, had been cured of malaria by an extract of this plant's bark (Lyons & Petrucelli, 1987). It was certainly imported into Europe after 1633 by the Jesuits. Malaria, the ague, was rife in many low-lying and marshy areas of Europe in the seventeenth century, and the Peruvian bark was an effective remedy. In 1763, the Rev. Edward Stone reported to the President of the Royal Society of London that an extract of the bark of the willow tree alleviated the ague. Thereafter this extract was used widely as an antipyretic, and by some unscrupulous physicians as a substitute for the expensive cinchona bark in the treatment of malaria. Of course, the salicylate which the willow bark contained had antipyretic actions but it did not contain the quinine found in the cinchona bark which was the proper substance to treat infection with the malarial parasite. The willow bark contains the glucoside salicin from which Piria (1838) first prepared salicylic acid. Other plants such as the birch (*Betula alba*) and cherry (*Prunus spinosa*) trees and the Gaultherias contain methylsalicylate. Gerland (1852) was the first to synthesize salicylic acid, though credit for this is usually given to Kolbe & Lautemann (1860). Acetylsalicylic acid was prepared by von Gerhardt in 1853 and this drug was introduced widely into medical practice by the Bayer company at the end of the nineteenth century as an analgesic, an anti-inflammatory compound and as an antipyretic. Other salicylates have also found wide usage in such illnesses as rheumatic fever and for superficial application in cases of

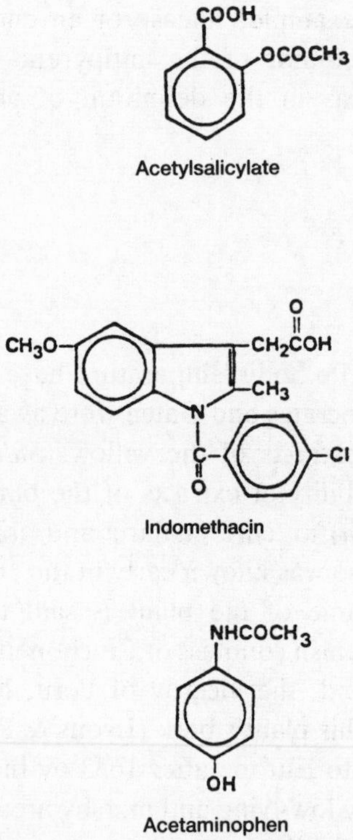

COOH
OCOCH₃

Acetylsalicylate

CH₃O—   CH₂COH
            CH₃
        N
        C—   —Cl
        O

Indomethacin

NHCOCH₃

OH

Acetaminophen

Fig. 7.1. The chemical formulae of the more commonly used antipyretics.

sprains and strains. A group of antipyretics derived from coal tar were discovered, starting in 1866, and these were derivatives of para-aminophenol, such as acetanilid and phenacetin. At about the same time, a group of pyrazolon compounds such as aminopyrine were also developed. These non-salicylate compounds, which were first used as antipyretics, also turned out to have analgesic and anti-inflammatory actions, though some had unpleasant side effects, such as agranulocytosis.

Some antipyretics currently in use

The commonest antipyretics used today are the salicylates (e.g., sodium salicylate and acetylsalicylic acid), indomethacin and the para-aminophenol derivative acetaminophen, all in a class known as non-steroidal antipyretics. These drugs also have anti-inflammatory and analgesic properties. The chemical formulae of the more commonly used antipyretics are given in Fig. 7.1. The original antimalarial drug, quinine, is occasionally used as an adjunct in treating malaria and is an antipyretic, but the mechanism of this latter action is not known. A full and most useful review of antipyretics and their actions can be found in Clark (1991).

Salicylate does enter the brain tissue and in afebrile rabbits receiving 300 mg sodium salicylate intravenously, the hypothalamic tissue concentration reaches 1.57 ± 0.35 mg/100 g and in febrile animals it reaches 1.76 ± 0.28 mg/100 g (Grundmann, 1969). Some antipyretics are lipophilic and this might in some circumstances assist them to cross the blood–brain barrier. The present evidence is that indomethacin does not cross the blood–brain barrier in significant amounts.

Concepts of the modes of action of antipyretics

The antipyretic actions of salicylates and other compounds remained a complete mystery until the 1970s. Many hypotheses were advanced earlier, but they lacked good evidence. Some, such as 'the antipyretic lowers the body temperature set point back to the normal level', were commonly stated in the textbooks but were no more than statements of the effect without shedding any light on the mechanisms. Other suggestions that the substances competed for pyrogen receptors in the thermoregulatory pathways, or that they adsorbed circulating pyrogen, were mooted but without evidence. Grundmann (1969) showed that salicylate does not inactivate endogenous pyrogen *in vitro* and that it does not prevent the release of endogenous pyrogen into the circulation. He tentatively suggested that salicylate might interfere with the passage of leucocyte pyrogen into the brain, but wisely commented that no positive evidence could be found for such a concept and that until a measurement of the passage or entry of leucocyte pyrogen into the brain, if any, this possibility could not properly be tested. In the light of present-day knowledge that labelled IL-1 cannot be traced within the brain following intravenous administration, it appears that Grundmann's suggestion is no longer tenable. The work of Cranston *et al.* (1970) in which both intravenous and icv salicylate were found to reduce an established fever, makes it unlikely that the concept of antipyresis by blocking the entry of endogenous pyrogen into the brain is valid.

Following the discoveries of Milton & Wendlandt (1971) that prostaglandins of the E series caused fever of very rapid onset when injected into the cerebral ventricles, and the subsequent work demonstrating the

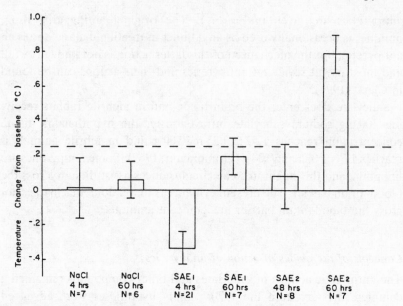

Fig. 7.2. Responses of newborn lambs to iv injection of $0.3 \, \mu g$ SAE or 0.9% NaCl at various times after birth. The subscript SAE_1 refers to first and SAE_2 to the second challenge. Bars and thin vertical lines represent means and twice the standard error of the means (SEM). The dashed line shows the upper limit of random temperature fluctuations. 'N' denotes the numbers of animals. (From Pittman, 1976.)

release of PGE_2 within the brain during fever (see Chapter 5), and the discovery by Vane (1971) that aspirin as well as other antipyretic and anti-inflammatory drugs inhibited the synthesis of prostaglandins, it has been postulated that antipyretic drugs reduce fever by inhibiting the formation of PGE_2 in the brain. That PGE injection into the appropriate brain regions does not always cause fever in animals that respond to endotoxins with fever (see Mitchell *et al.*, 1986) suggests that the prostaglandin synthesis inhibition may not be the only mode of action of antipyretics. The experimental evidence is further confused by the observations of Alexander *et al.* (1989) that salicylate infusions into the VSA block the febrile response to PGE_1 given into the cerebral ventricles. A similar reduction in PGE induced fever was found using indomethacin (Fyda *et al.*, 1989). While these observations do not mitigate against PGE as a component of the febrile process, they do indicate a possible action of two commonly used antipyretics other than inhibition of PGE synthesis. The evidence to date must compel acceptance of inhibition of PGE synthesis as one important mechanism of antipyretic action, but other actions of commonly used antipyretics to modulate the several phases of fever resulting from natural infections or experimentally administered pyrogens cannot be excluded. Such actions could include competitive antagonism at the IL-1, or other pyrogenic cytokine receptor, the release of an endogenous antipyretic substance which does not act through PGE synthesis inhibition or a direct action on the discharge rate of the neurons controlling the apparent set point or on the efferent pathways responsible for raising the body temperature.

The concept of endogenous antipyresis

At a Ciba Foundation symposium on pyrogens and fever (Wolstenholme & Birch, 1971), during an informal discussion, both M. Landy and W. I. Cranston raised the question as to whether the newborn animal would be able to mount a fever in response to infection or administration of bacterial pyrogen or whether the animal's macrophages need priming in order to elaborate and release endogenous pyrogen. I raised this problem in our laboratory when I returned to Calgary and work started on it soon after in the PhD studies of Q. J. Pittman. He decided to study the newborn lamb because that animal is born with a very mature thermoregulatory system which has all of the physiological or autonomic mechanisms for thermoregulation in place at birth. Pittman (1976) showed that the sheep foetus, while still *in utero*, responded to intravenous endotoxin with a fall in circulating white cell count but with no change in core temperature. The transitory leucopaenia is a characteristic response to iv endotoxin in the adult. Lambs were given intravenous endotoxin in doses adequate to induce fever in the adult sheep at various times after birth. An injection of endotoxin at four hours or a first injection at 60 hours after birth failed to cause fever, but if lambs which had received endotoxin at four hours after delivery were given a second dose at 60 hours post-partum they did respond with fever (Fig. 7.2). There appeared to be a necessary sensitization process after birth in order to obtain a fever response. The sensitization could be produced by various antigenically different exogenous substances, and could also be induced by giving endotoxin intravenously *in utero* during the final few days of gestation. Of interest also was Pittman's finding that the newborn lamb, even when able to respond to intravenous pyrogen with fever, did not get fever in response to micro-injection of prostaglandins into the hypothalamus or cerebral ventricles.

Following these observations, Kasting observed the body temperature responses to intravenous endotoxin in newborn lambs and at various times pre- and post-partum (Kasting, 1980). In the experiments on newborn lambs Kasting gave bacterial pyrogen intravenously (30 μg as compared to 0.3 μg used by Pittman) and found that at four hours after birth the lambs experienced a hypothermia of approximately 0.5°C, and at 30 hours after delivery they had fevers of the same magnitude as control lambs of six-days-old or adult ewes. Intravenous administration of sheep endogenous pyrogen gave the same pattern of response. The hypothermia was accompanied by some symptoms of distress. It would appear that the need for sensitization can be bypassed by using much larger (100 fold) doses of endotoxin. While the response of the 30-hour-old lambs to the low dose of endotoxin after an initial dose at four hours post-partum still suggests a sensitization process, the induction of fever in non-sensitized lambs of 30 hours post-partum with the high dose of endotoxin suggests the possibility of a circulating antipyretic in the immediate post-partum period.

The ewes were found to get progressively smaller fevers from the fourth day pre-partum to between 5 and 32 hours post-partum. Appropriate experimental design eliminated tolerance to the pyrogen as a factor. Kasting also found that the leucocytes of pregnant ewes taken at a time when the animals were resistant to endotoxin and from foetal lambs were able to produce endogenous pyrogen. From these early experiments Kasting concluded that fever in the ewe and newborn lamb can be suppressed close to term and shortly after delivery by some endogenously produced substance to which he gave the term endogenous antipyretic.

There have been reports contrary to the findings of Kasting and his colleagues. Heap *et al*. (1981), and Blatteis *et al*. (1988) were unable to demonstrate suppression of fever close to term in the sheep. However, Goelst *et al*. (1992) did a study on Dorper sheep in which the same ewes were used to test the response to bacterial pyrogens pre- and post-partum. They were able to confirm Kasting's findings of reduced fever responses to Gram-negative endotoxin, and to show that the fall in serum iron which normally accompanies fever was only suppressed in the immediate pre-partum period. However, there was no suppression of fever or serum iron depression either pre- or post-partum after administration of *Staphylococcus aureus* cell walls. So it looked as though the response to Gram-negative endotoxin is suppressed in the peripar-

Pillay *et al*. (1994) report a rise in levels of IT-receptor antagonist in the plasma of neonates and near term women, adding another means of fever suppression at term.

tum, but that an intact temperature-raising mechanism remains. The differences between others who did not observe fever suppression in the peripartum and Kasting may lie in the strain of sheep used, or the failure to follow the responses longitudinally in the sheep. Zeisberger *et al.* (1981) found fever suppression in the guinea-pig in the peripartum.

The possible value of an endogenous antipyretic system activated in the immediate pre- and post-partum periods has been discussed (Veale *et al.*, 1981), and the possibilities are intriguing but speculative. The proper development and action of lung surfactant would be impaired at febrile temperatures; the relative hypoxia of the foetal brain would increase with a rise in the maternal and hence the foetal temperature; possibly the enhancing effect of a rise in temperature on the maternal immune system could enable the mother to mount immunological defences against the foetus at a time when the placental barrier begins to be less firm; and there could be foetal damage engendered by a high temperature in other ways. Bonding between the ewe and the lamb could be impaired by fever experienced by either.

Putative peptide mediators of endogenous antipyresis

Arginine vasopressin as an endogenous antipyretic

The evidence
A study of the literature indicated that circulating AVP rose close to term but the evidence was controversial (Alexander *et al.*, 1974; Stark *et al.*, 1979). Also, AVP containing neurons in the hypothalamus and elsewhere in the brain had been demonstrated (Buijs *et al.*, 1978; Sofroniew & Weindl, 1978; Weindl & Sofroniew, 1985). AVP circulating in the blood was shown not to have an antipyretic action (Cooper *et al.*, 1979). Using stereotaxic techniques and push–pull perfusion, AVP was applied to various brain regions during fever to seek for a location in which it might suppress fever in the sheep. One region was found (Kasting, 1980) in the ventral septum. It was 2–3 mm anterior to the anterior commissure and close to the diagonal band of Broca. Perfusion of this region with sucrose solution (an inert medium used to control the perfusate osmolarity) was without effect on fever induced by bacterial endotoxin. However, when the perfusate contained AVP (4.0 μg/ml) and was administered in the VSA at 40 μl/min, fever was markedly reduced (Fig. 7.3). There was a linear negative correlation between the concentration of AVP in the perfusate and the fever response. AVP was measured in

perfusates from the septal area during pyrogen-induced fevers and was found to be negatively related to the fever height. There was one precise locus in which AVP had an antipyretic action. AVP perfused within the ventral septum was without effect on the body temperature of the afebrile animal. In other loci, Banet & Wieland (1985) found effects of AVP on thermoregulation in the rat. In the lateral septum it reduced the increased heat production resulting from preoptic cooling, or to cold exposure, but did not alter thermoregulation at the upper end of thermoneutrality, and the authors suggested that the body temperature set point was not altered. This observation underlines the differences in actions of AVP in different loci and the need for precise localization of the point of application of the peptide in studies of endogenous antipyresis.

The antipyretic action of AVP within the brain has been tested in species other than the sheep. Ruwe *et al.* (1985) found that AVP perfused through the ventral septal area of the rat suppressed the fever caused by icv administration of PGE_2. AVP given into the lateral septal area did not reduce PGE-induced fever. It is interesting that they also found a locus at which PGE_2 evoked fever which was close to the site at which AVP was antipyretic. Naylor *et al.* (1985) perfused the ventral septal area of the rabbit with AVP and found that it suppressed fever due to intravenous administration of endotoxin (Fig. 7.4). AVP infused into a lateral cerebral ventricle did not reduce endotoxin fever. In this respect it is interesting that Harvey Cushing (1931) did report a marked fall in the body temperature of a patient in whom a crude vasopressin-containing preparation (pituitrin) was administered into a cerebral ventricle. Bernadini *et al.* (1983) had injected AVP into the lateral septum in the rabbit and found that it did not reduce fever, but their extrapolation to the statement that AVP is not antipyretic in the rabbit was not justified because they did not use the correct locus for injection. Zeisberger (1989) demonstrated that AVP micro-infused in very small amounts into the ventral septum of guinea-pigs attenuated fever. Thus the same antipyretic response to intraseptal administration of AVP is found to occur in four species, and the locus of its antipyretic action is the same in all of them.

Haemorrhage is a potent stimulus for the release of AVP into the csf and the blood. Kasting *et al.* (1981) found that rapid removal of 20% of the estimated circulating blood volume greatly reduced the fever response to intravenous endotoxin, and it was likely that the reduced fevers were due to intracerebral release of AVP. It is interesting that

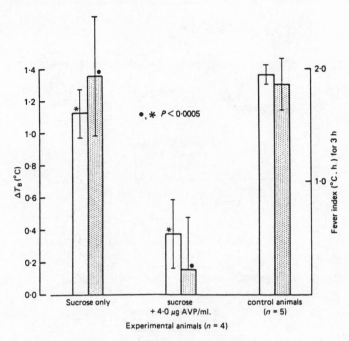

Fig. 7.3. Vertical bars represent the maximum fever height (open bars) during 200 min and the 3 h fever index (°C h) (stippled bars) in experimental animals following push–pull perfusion (40 μl/min) with sucrose only in the septal area, and with sucrose plus 4.0 μg AVP/ml in the same sites. Fever height and fever index were both significantly decreased when AVP was added to sucrose. The bars on the right represent the fever height and fever index in control (unoperated) animals. Vertical lines represent mean ± S.E. of mean. (From Cooper *et al.*, 1979.)

reduced 'fever heat' was noted by the ancient physicians to follow deliberate haemorrhage in the days of blood letting (Wunderlich, 1871).

Another approach to the investigation of AVP as an endogenous antipyretic has been to block or reduce the action of the peptide within the septum and to record the effect of this on fever. Malkinson *et al.* (1987) perfused the ventral septum of the rabbit with a highly specific antibody to AVP and observed the effect on fever induced by intravenous endotoxin. They showed that the perfusions were in the correct locus because AVP added to the perfusing medium reduced the fever. Addition of the AVP antibody to perfusing fluid resulted in greatly enhanced fevers which implied that neutralizing the endogenously released AVP resulted in greater fevers and thus the local release of AVP was important in restraining the fever process. In the periphery there

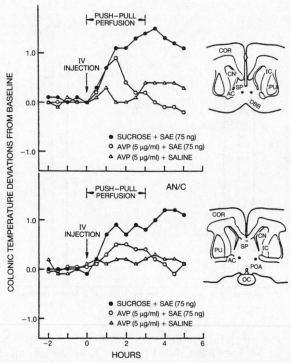

Fig. 7.4. Colonic temperature in deviations from baseline (°C) in two rabbits. AVP at a concentration of 5.0 μg/ml (open circles) or the vehicle solution alone (sucrose; closed circles) was perfused into the VSA immediately prior to and for 3.0 hr after an iv injection of SAE (75 ng) at time zero. Perfusion of AVP after an iv injection of saline (open triangles) was without effect on resting body temperature. Loci of perfusions are indicated by closed circles on the histological insets. Abbreviations: AC – anterior commissure; CN – caudate nucleus; COR – cortex; DBB – diagonal band of broca; IC – internal capsule; OC – optic chiasm; POA – preoptic area; PU – putamen; SP – septum pellucidum. (From Naylor *et al.*, 1985.)

are several AVP receptor types including the V_1 (the vasopressor receptor) and the V_2 (the antidiuretic receptor). Antagonists to these two have been injected into the ventral septal area of the rat before IL-1 was given into a lateral cerebral ventricle (Cooper *et al.*, 1987). Saline injected into the ventral septal area did not attenuate IL-1 fever. However, when the vasopressin V_1 antagonist, d(CH$_2$)$_5$Tyr(Me)AVP (200–400 pmol), was injected into the ventral septal area 15 min before human purified IL-1 (hpIL-1) was fed into a lateral cerebral ventricle by gravity (dose: 20 units in 20 μl saline), the fever was enhanced in a dose-related way (Figs. 7.5 a & b). Injection of the V_1 antagonist into

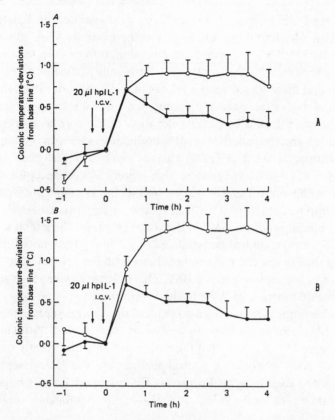

Fig. 7.5. (A) mean temperature response ($\pm$ S.E. of mean) to the icv infusion of hpIL-1 (20 units). 15 min prior to this, either 1.0 μl saline ($\bullet$, n = 6) or 200 pmol of the vasopressin V_1 antagonist d(CH$_2$)$_5$Tyr(Me)AVP (O, n = 6) were injected bilaterally into the VSA (first arrow). (B) mean temperature response ($\pm$ S.E. of mean) to the icv infusion of hpIL-1 (20 units). 15 min prior to this, either 1.0 μl saline ($\bullet$, n = 7) or 400 pmol of the vasopressin V_1 antagonist d(CH$_2$)$_5$Tyr(Me)AVP (O, n = 7), were injected bilaterally into the VSA (first arrow). (From Cooper *et al.*, 1987.)

the ventral septal area, or of the saline vehicle, was without effect on the afebrile rat's temperature. The vasopressin V_2 antagonist [d(CH$_2$)$_5$-D-ValVAVP] was also injected into the ventral septal area under the same circumstances and did not alter the magnitude or time course of the IL-1 fever. The results of these experiments are not only consistent with the notion of an antipyretic action of AVP within the ventral septum but suggest that the AVP receptor is similar, or identical, to the peripheral V_1 receptor. Reduction of body temperature consistent with release of AVP into the ventral septum of the urethane anaesthetized rat during PGE$_1$-induced fever has been demonstrated by Landgraf *et al.* (1990), who found that the fever was increased by VSA administration of the AVP-V$_1$ antagonist. Passive alteration of core temperature was not modified by the antagonist. Push–pull perfusion of the VSA showed that there was increased release of AVP only after PGE-induced fever and not after passively raising the animal's temperature, but oxytocin was released by passive elevation of the core temperature.

Location and characterization of subcellular vasopressin binding sites, using tritium labelled AVP, in various brain loci has been studied (Poulin *et al.*, 1988). They found high affinity V$_1$-like receptor sites in the rat in the ventral septal area as well as the lateral septum and the hippocampus. Szot *et al.* (1990) have also, using tritiated AVP, found specific binding sites for AVP in the ventral septum, the lateral septum, the BST and the central amygdala among others. They noted that the binding sites in the cell membranes showed similar selectivity to the V$_1$ receptor in the septum and the BST. This is further evidence in support of a specific function of AVP in the ventral septum.

Another approach has been to deplete the ventral septal area of its vasopressin content, in rats, by castration early in life. Pittman *et al.* (1988) were able to show that their castrated rats had greatly depleted stores of AVP in both the ventral septum and the lateral septum as compared to sham castrated controls. The castrated animals responded to icv doses of both PGE$_1$ and IL-1 with significantly enhanced fevers.

There is good immunohistological evidence for involvement of AVP in hypothalamic and septal responses to pyrogens in both the non-pregnant and pregnant guinea-pig. Merker *et al.* (1980) were able to show denser immunoreactivity for central AVP neuron projections, both in septal areas and the paraventricular nuclei, in the brains of near term pregnant and foetal guinea-pigs and in early neonates. These experiments revealed that there was an increased amount of vasopressin immunoreactive material in the medial region of the hypothalamic paraventricular nucleus and in terminals and preterminals in the lateral septum and also the amygdala. Zeisberger *et al.* (1983) showed that immunoreactivity for AVP increased in fibres projecting from the hypothalamus to the septum during fever. Increased immunoreactivity for AVP was found (Cooper *et al.*, 1988) in the medial paraventricular nucleus and in terminals in the lateral septum and amygdala of the guinea-pig following repeated injections and tolerance to the synthetic pyrogen Poly I:Poly C (a double-stranded synthetic polynucleotide).

The main sources of AVP released in the septum appear to be neurons derived from PVN and the BST. The preponderance of one source or another varies with the species. In the rat the main region of origin of septal neurons containing AVP is the BST and in the guinea-pig the PVN and also the supraoptic nucleus (Zeisberger, 1991). Using electrophysiological methods, neurons have been identified in the ventral septal area of the rat which receive afferent impulses from the BST and the PVN (Disturnal *et al.*, 1985, 1986). The regions of origin of these neurons are known to have AVP-containing neurons and were mostly connected with thermosensitive units which responded to thermal stimulation of the scrotal skin. Neurons projecting to the VSA from the PVN when stimulated electrically caused orthodromic inhibition of most thermosensitive VSA thermosensitive units; and from the BST inhibition of warm sensitive and excitation of cold sensitive units. It is of great interest that there are IL-1β containing neurons in the BST (Lechan *et al.*, 1990). Recently, Wilkinson *et al.* (1993) have demonstrated that human recombinant IL-1 applied by electrophoresis or micro-injection within the BST in urethane anaesthetized rats caused prolonged excitation of 24% of BST cells studied. Iontophoresis of salicylate at the same locus blocked or attenuated the excitation suggesting an involvement of prostaglandin in the excitatory process. This work suggests a possible mechanism, via release of IL-1 within the BST, in the release of the endogenous antipyretic AVP in the ventral septum. Afferents to the VSA were also found derived from the amygdala, a region known to have some AVP neurons that project from the hypothalamus. A small proportion of single units in the BST have been found to increase their firing rate during fever caused by icv administration of PGE (Mathieson *et al.*, 1989). Disturnal *et al.* (1987) also studied the effect of AVP applied by micro-iontophoresis on to glutamate excited neurons and spontaneously active neurons. AVP was shown to reduce the activity of most glutamate excited units and this AVP induced inhibition was reversed by application of the AVP-V_1 blocker. This combined with the demonstration of inhibitory input from both the BST and PVN could suggest one possible mode of action of AVP in reducing the fever drive.

Electrical stimulation of the bed nucleus of the stria terminalis of the rat reduces fever induced by intraventricular PGE_1, and the fever suppression is abolished by micro-injection of the V_1 receptor antagonist into the VSA (Naylor *et al.*, 1988). This provides further evidence for release of AVP in the VSA from neurons derived from the BST in the rat. A very recent study (Wilkinson *et al.*, 1994) showed that IL-1β infused into the BST caused fever but also led to increased release of AVP into the VSA; this release was independent of the core temperature *per se*. The presence of IL-1 in neurons in the BST has been clearly demonstrated (Breder *et al.*, 1988; Lechan *et al.*, 1990; Molenaar *et al.*, 1993). The functions of these neurons have not yet been determined. It is possible that some of them could release IL-1 in response to the events which follow the peripheral administration of endotoxin or in fever causing disease. This release could possibly be a step in engendering the release of AVP as an antipyretic feedback system in addition to being a determinant, possibly not the main one, of the rise in core temperature. Such a tentative suggestion can be inferred from the work of Wilkinson *et al.* (1994) who also suggest that the source of some IL-1 containing neurons in the BST could be the paraventricular nucleus.

Lesions produced by kainic acid, which is an analogue of glutamate, destroy cell somata and dendrites while not affecting the neurons of passage. Kainic acid was injected into the ventral septal area (Martin *et al.*, 1988) and the rats experienced enhanced fevers. These experiments again emphasize the importance of the VSA in the modulation of fever.

With the knowledge of the presence of AVP-containing neurons in the amygdala and the demonstrated connections between the amygdala and the VSA, experiments were undertaken to explore a possible role for AVP in the amygdala in endogenous antipyresis (Federico *et al.*, 1992 a,b,c). Earlier, Kasting & Martin (1983) had shown that AVP levels in the amygdala fell during endotoxin induced fever. Others had found increased immunoreactivity for AVP in terminals in the amygdala during fever and at term in guinea-pigs (Zeisberger *et al.*, 1983, 1986). The studies of Federico *et al.* (1992b) were carried out on urethane anaesthetized rats. AVP was applied to the medial amygdaloid nucleus by push–pull perfusion and its effect on fever induced by icv PGE$_1$ was recorded. AVP given 6.5 μg/ml at 16 μl/min greatly reduced the PGE fever (Fig. 7.6). Further to this study, Federico *et al.* (1992c) injected the AVP-V$_1$ (strictly the V$_{1a}$) receptor antagonist and found that it antagonized the antipyretic action of AVP micro-injected into the medial amygdaloid nucleus. The antipyretic action of locally applied AVP in the amygdala is significant but less than that when AVP is applied within the VSA. They were not able to confirm the blocking of *endogenously* released AVP as having a major effect on fever, but results gained in their experimental design do not rule out a possible role for the

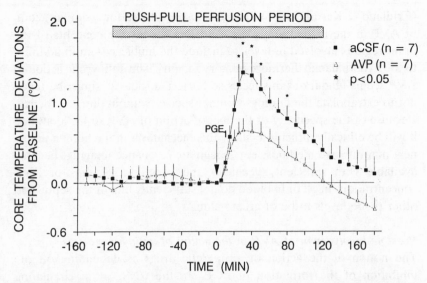

Fig. 7.6. Mean (± S.E.M.) changes in colonic temperature in response to the icv injection of PGE$_1$ during the perfusion of aCSF (filled squares) or AVP (open triangles) within the MEA (* < 0.05). (From Federico *et al.*, 1992b.)

amygdala in endogenous antipyresis or in the development of tolerance to pyrogens.

Cooper *et al.* (1979) found that AVP infused intravenously into sheep in amounts of 0.24, 2.4 or 24.0 μg/200 min, did not significantly reduce the fever induced by bacterial pyrogen given iv. Thus, the action of AVP as an endogenous antipyretic appeared to be confined to the CNS release. However, Milton *et al.* (1993b) have studied the action of AVP given peripherally on fever produced by the synthetic pyrogen PolyI:Poly C. They found that the AVP-V$_1$ receptor antagonist, administered 5 min before the pyrogen significantly antagonized the fever. It also reduced the circulating level of immunoreactive PGE$_2$. The pyrogen used induces TNF$_\alpha$ which is an endogenous pyrogen, and the difference between these results and those of Cooper *et al.* (1979) may lie in the different cytokine pathway evoked peripherally. The results of Milton *et al.* (1993b) suggest that in their paradigm the peripheral antipyretic action of AVP is via actions of PGE$_2$.

The evidence presented in the section above supporting a modulatory role for AVP in fever, acting through the ventral septal area, is extensive and very powerful. Recent work indicates an antipyretic role for AVP not only in artificial fever but also in fever due to bacterial infection

(Cridland & Kasting, 1992). There is also evidence for a similar action of AVP in the medial amygdala, and this widens the concepts of the brain regions involved in fever to include the limbic system in addition to the hypothalamic thermoregulatory regions. The antipyretic action of AVP seems ubiquitous in species so far tested, but care must be taken not to extrapolate the findings to other species without direct evidence. Because of the specificity of the loci of action of AVP so far identified it will be ethically difficult to study this mechanism in the human unless new non-invasive methods, e.g., magnetic resonance imaging, become available with sufficient specificity and precision. Studies of AVP concentrations in csf or in blood do not sufficiently mirror the septal and other tissue levels to be of great value.

Possible involvement of AVP in the action of antipyretic drugs
The notion of the action of antipyretic drugs as depending on the inhibition of the formation of PGE_2 in the CNS, or in circulating macrophages has much evidence to support it. It has been necessary, however, to test the hypothesis that other mechanisms of action of antipyretics could be available in the brain. Alexander *et al.* (1989) studied the effect of infusing sodium salicylate into the ventral septal area of the rat brain on fever induced by icv administration of PGE_1. At 50 or 100 μg/ml, infused at the rate of 1 μl/h, the salicylate suppressed the PGE_1-induced fever. Simultaneous infusion of salicylate with either AVP antiserum or AVP antagonist resulted in an unaltered PGE_1 fever. Thus salicylate is able to block the febrogenic action of PGE_1, as well as to inhibit its production through an action in the ventral septum probably via vasopressin release. Wilkinson & Kasting (1990b) were able to show that the antipyretic action of salicylate in the rat ventral septum could be blocked by $AVP-V_1$ receptor blockade, in endotoxin-induced fever. Acetaminophen antipyresis, elicited in the VSA, was not altered by VSA administration of the $AVP-V_1$ blocker. A study by Fyda *et al.* (1990) showed that both salicylate and AVP infused into the ventral septal area of the Brattleboro rat reduced fever caused by icv administration of PGE_1. This strain of rat is said to be devoid of AVP in cerebral neurons as well as peripherally. However, there is evidence for the existence of AVP receptors in the Brattleboro rat brain (Ravid *et al.*, 1986), and there is some evidence for the presence of vasopressin associated glycopeptide in the brain and periphery of this type of rat. So, the possibility still exists that the application of AVP in the septum of the Brattleboro rat produces antipyresis by acting on vasopressin

receptors there, and that there could be enough endogenous vasopressin in the septal area to mediate the salicylate antipyresis. An alternative explanation would be that the salicylate acted through another peptide mediator such as α-MSH, but to date there is no evidence for this.

A possible role for vasopressin in pyrogen tolerance
It has long been known that repeated daily injections of bacterial pyrogens induce a state of tolerance in the animal. This is manifest as a reduced fever response to a given dose of pyrogen assessed as a lower fever index (the area under the temperature rise and fall curve) and this is due mainly to a reduction in the second peak of fever (Pickering, 1961). The tolerance remains for about three weeks after cessation of the pyrogen administration. The tolerance does not seem to be a simple immune response since it does not parallel the blood titre of immune bodies, and there is cross-tolerance even when there is no cross immunity if different bacterial sources are used. A tolerant animal always gets a minimal fever in response to pyrogen injection even after as many as 24 daily injections (Whittet, 1980; Fig. 7.7). There is evidence that part of the mechanism of tolerance is peripheral to the CNS. In a tolerant animal, administration of endogenous pyrogen causes fever (Bennet & Beeson, 1953b). Bacterial pyrogen labelled with ^{131}I is cleared from the circulation in two phases, about 80% in the first 7–12 min after injection and the remainder very slowly. The initial rapid clearance from the rabbit circulation is more rapid in tolerant than in non-tolerant animals (Cooper & Cranston, 1963). The slow clearance is similar in both sets of animals, an observation which agrees with that of two other studies using ^{51}Cr-labelled pyrogen in rabbits and ^{32}P-labelled pyrogen in mice and guinea-pigs (Rowley *et al.*, 1956; Braude *et al.*, 1958); but Braude *et al.* (1958) did not find an accelerated clearance in the first phase while Rowley *et al.* (1956) did. Administration of Indian ink (Beeson, 1947) or thorotrast (colloidal thorium dioxide) (Beeson, 1947; Whittet, 1980; Fig. 7.7), both of which are said to block the cells of the RES, prior to pyrogen injection restores the fever to pre-tolerance levels. The Indian ink result may well have been in part due to induction of tolerance by another endotoxin, present in the ink, to which the animal was not already tolerant (Landy, 1971), and the effect of thorotrast may have been the result of increasing the sensitivity to endotoxin, and possibly to enhancing opsonic factors in the blood which are in part responsible for pyrogen clearance (Snell, 1971). Thorotrast itself also can cause fever in both tolerant and naïve rabbits

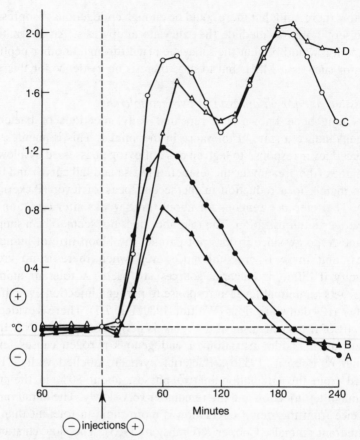

Fig. 7.7. Abolition of tolerance to SAE pyrogen and to London tap water by
iv injection of colloidal thorium dioxide.
A – SAE pyrogen   (50 ng/kg) day 23
B – Sterile London tap water (10 ml/kg) day 23
C – SAE pyrogen   (50 ng/kg) day 24 +thorium
D – Sterile London tap water (10 ml/kg) day 24 +thorium
(From Whittet, 1980.)

and it may not abolish more than a small proportion of tolerance activity
(Greisman *et al.*, 1963). So while there is evidence for extracerebral
mechanisms involved in tolerance to pyrogens, much of which is
controversial, there is new information which may implicate the endogenous antipyretic system in development of tolerance. Cooper *et al.*
(1988) found increased immunoreactivity for AVP in the septum in
guinea-pigs made tolerant to Poly I:Poly C. Wilkinson & Kasting
(1990a) demonstrated that administration of the AVP-V_1 receptor

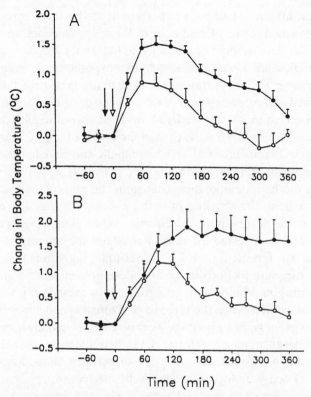

Fig. 7.8. Mean change ± SE in body temperature (°C) in response to intravenous endotoxin (open arrow) in endotoxin-tolerant rats; 15 min before this, 0.5 μl of saline (open circles) or V_1 antagonist [d(CH$_2$)$_5$Tyr(Me)]AVP (closed circles) was bilaterally injected into VSA (closed arrow). (A) effect of 0.43 nmol V_1 antagonist or saline administered bilaterally within VSA on body temperature response to endotoxin. Mean base-line body temperatures were saline (VSA) + endotoxin, 37.73 ± 0.18 °C (n = 8); 0.43 nmol V_1 antagonist (VSA) + endotoxin, 37.41 ± 0.11 °C (n = 8). (B) effect of 4.3 nmol V_1 antagonist or saline administered within VSA on body temperature response to endotoxin. Mean base-line body temperatures were saline (VSA) + endotoxin, 37.37 ± 0.08 °C (n = 6); 4.3 nmol V_1 antagonist (VSA) + endotoxin, 37.32 ± 0.09 °C (n = 6). (From Wilkinson & Kasting, 1990a.)

antagonist in the ventral septal area of the endotoxin-tolerant rat, enhanced the fever response to further doses of the pyrogen in a dose-dependent manner (Fig. 7.8). The AVP-V_2 receptor antagonist was without effect. These results could be construed as either suggesting that the AVP antipyretic system is involved in the mechanism of tolerance or that the AVP-V_1 antagonist, which given into the VSA enhances fever, was merely enhancing the portion of the bacterial pyrogen fever which remained in the tolerant animal. While the evidence for a role for AVP in the development of tolerance to bacterial pyrogen is available, more studies are needed to clinch the hypothesis. A recent study (Zeisberger et al., 1994), raised the probability that three factors may be involved in the development of tolerance to endotoxin, namely, more rapid inactivation of the bacterial pyrogen, down-regulation of the cytokine response (TNF & IL-6)[*] and the action of a central antipyretic mechanism. Plasma levels of TNF rise rapidly and peak in the first hour after endotoxin administration, and the plasma IL-6 activity rises and parallels the body temperature change in the non-tolerant animal. In tolerant animals the activities of both cytokines decreased in a manner parallel to the decreased fever response. When guinea-pigs were made tolerant and then rested for three weeks and the process of inducing tolerance was repeated, it took a shorter time, suggesting that previous pyrogen exposure had accelerated the development of tolerance. Continuous infusion of endotoxin into guinea-pigs caused only a small rise in core temperature over the three days of infusion and none thereafter, and in pregnant guinea-pigs there were no changes in body temperature. The non-pregnant animals clearly developed tolerance after three days and the pregnant ones were resistant to pyrogen altogether, possibly because of active endogenous antipyretic mechanisms.

A most interesting and potentially clinically important study by Wilkinson & Pittman (1994) has dealt with the response of pyrogen-tolerant animals, following endotoxin injection, to intra-peritoneal administration of the antipyretic drug indomethacin. Tolerant eight-week-old rats who were given indomethacin two hours after bacterial pyrogen injection developed a profound and dose-dependent hypothermia, and there was a 41% mortality rate within 24 hours. Neither the severe hypothermia nor the high mortality were found to occur in 20-week tolerant animals. The low body temperatures and the high death rates were prevented by giving the AVP-V_1 receptor antagonist into the VSA. These results suggest that AVP release played a major role in the deleterious responses to indomethacin in juvenile rats and, although pathological correlates have not yet been demonstrated, might lead to an animal model for the study of Reye's syndrome.

*Since the manuscript was finished, information has been published which indicates both TNF-like and IL-1-like activities in guinea-pig plasma, released in response to bacterial pyrogen, diminish as tolerance to the pyrogen develops (Roth et al., 1994).

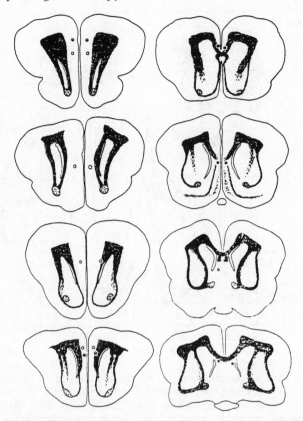

Fig. 7.9. Central sites of cannula placements of animals that had antipyretic responses to α-MSH (●) and those that did not (○). (◑) indicates animals responding 50% of the time. Most of the positive placements were in the septal region; however, two animals with placements rostral to the septum responded to α-MSH. Tissue of two animals that did not respond was lost in processing. Rostral-caudal sequence: left column, from top to bottom, continued in right column. (From Glyn-Ballinger *et al.*, 1983.)

α-MSH as an endogenous antipyretic

Lipton & Glyn (1980) found that a number of peptides injected into the cerebral ventricles altered body temperature in rabbits and among these, α-MSH and ACTH induced dose dependent falls in core temperature. Others, such as oxytocin, vasopressin and glucagon, caused increases in body temperature. Samson *et al.* (1981) showed that fever raised the levels of α-MSH in the septal region of rabbits. Also, Glyn & Lipton (1981) showed that doses of α-MSH which were insufficient to affect normal core temperature, reduced fever when given centrally. Glyn-

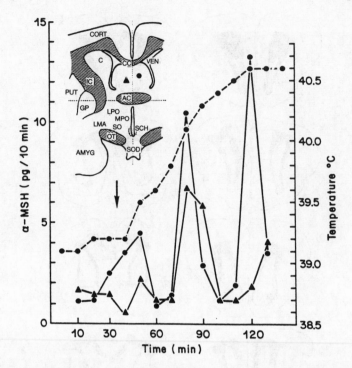

Fig. 7.10. α-Melanocyte-stimulating hormone (α-MSH) concentration of push–pull perfusate (solid lines) sampled every 10 min in one rabbit. IL-1 was injected intravenously at arrow. Dashed line, body temperature. Both discrete (filled circles, response mainly confined to one 10-min period, see peaks at 80 and 120 min) and continuous or repeated (filled triangles, 70–100 min) patterns of release are represented. (From Bell & Lipton, 1987.)

Ballinger *et al.* (1983) identified a region in the lateral septum in which injected α-MSH could reduce fever caused by leucocyte pyrogen in the rabbit (Fig. 7.9). Bell & Lipton (1987) demonstrated pulsatile release of α-MSH from the lateral septum during fever induced by IL-1 in the rabbit (Fig. 7.10), and the release was greatest during the chill phase of fever. Intravenous α-MSH has also been shown to reduce fever in the squirrel monkey (*Saimiri sciureus*) (Shih & Lipton, 1985) and it also lowers fever in the guinea-pig (Kandasamy & Williams, 1984), but apparently not in the cat (Rezvani *et al.*, 1986). The α-MSH- containing neurons projecting to the lateral septum are derived mainly from the arcuate nucleus. These can be depleted of their α-MSH content by treating the rat as a neonate with MSG. Martin *et al.* (1990) have shown that such MSG treated rats, the α-MSH depletion in which was verified, had exaggerated fevers in response to PGE_1 and IL-1. These observations are consistent with the notion that α-MSH is an endogenous antipyretic. Shih *et al.* (1986) found that administration of an α-MSH antiserum into the third cerebral ventricle markedly enhanced fever. It is also of great interest that intragastric administration of α-MSH reduces fever, induced by intravenous leucocyte pyrogen, in the rabbit and they also found that the older animals were more sensitive to the antipyretic effect of α-MSH than were younger ones (Lipton & Murphy, 1983). This could be part of the mechanism of reduced fever response known to occur (Ferguson *et al.*, 1981) in older animals. Intravenous α-MSH attenuated the fever response to bacterial pyrogen, rabbit endogenous pyrogen, $TNF\alpha$, and IL-1β as well as reducing the plasma PGE_2 levels which had been raised by the pyrogen (Davidson *et al.*, 1992). However, α-MSH did not alter the fever produced by icv administration of PGE_2. The authors suggested that the antipyretic action of α-MSH in these experiments could have been by preventing synthesis of PGE_2 by acting on the function or release of pyrogenic cytokines by bacterial pyrogen.

Thus the evidence strongly supports the concept of α-MSH as an endogenous antipyretic both within the brain and peripherally. Less is known, at the time of writing, about the intracerebral receptor binding or electrophysiological correlates of α-MSH than those of AVP, and these will form exciting studies in the future.

The roles of CRF in fever and fever inhibition
There is controversy over the 'central' action of CRF as a fever modulator. Bernadini *et al.* (1984) micro-injected CRF into the third ventricle in the rabbit in doses of 0.5–2.5 μg and observed a dose-related reduction of fever induced by iv leucocyte pyrogen. They found that iv CRF, which in other species had been shown to release ACTH and corticosteroids, did not cause a reduction of fever. They surmised, however, that icv CRF could have been more effective in releasing ACTH and α-MSH centrally. These substances could then have acted as antipyretics. Opp *et al.* (1989) found that IL-1 administration caused a rise in brain temperature, i.e., a fever, and that 0.1–0.5 μg CRF reduced this fever after a long delay. On the other hand Rothwell (1989) reported experiments done in rats in which 50 ng of IL-1β given icv caused fever and a rise in oxygen consumption which was mainly due to increased BAT activity. Prior injection of a CRF receptor antagonist [helical CRF(9-41)] at a dose of 254μg prevented or markedly attenuated

the fever and the rise in oxygen consumption. The fever responses were also inhibited by prior administration of an antibody to CRF. However, the fevers induced by ip endotoxin, TNFα, or icv PGE$_2$ were not blocked by the CRF antagonist. So in this work it seems as though the IL-1β fever inducing pathway may use a CRF link, but the other three pyrogens act through a pathway not requiring CRF. In addition Rothwell (1989) showed that, in mice, CRF (4 μg given icv) caused a rise in metabolic rate which was not blocked by the cyclo-oxygenase inhibitor, ibuprofen, given ip at a dose of 5 mg/kg. Thus this action was apparently not PGE$_2$ mediated. Rothwell (1990) also found that both PGE$_2$ and PGF$_{2\alpha}$ given icv caused fever and a rise in oxygen uptake in rats. CRF did likewise. However, CRF + PGE$_2$ fever responses were additive whereas CRF + PGF$_{2\alpha}$ were not. The CRF receptor antagonist inhibited the effects of PGF$_{2\alpha}$ but not those caused by PGE$_2$. It would seem from this that PGF$_{2\alpha}$ is involved in IL-1β-induced fever, which has been shown probably to require CRF for its induction. Further work by Rothwell (1993) would indicate that the actions in the brain of IL-6 depend on CRF, and that there are many possible biochemical pathways in the brain which come into play in a way dependent on how the particular pyrogenic cytokine is acting.

This seems a good place at which to discuss the problems inherent in icv administration of substances and some other technical difficulties. Administration icv often leads to results which are contradictory and are difficult to explain. The amount injected compared to the volume of the ventricle used, the volume flow of csf and the concentration reaching the loci of action of the substance, can all influence the outcome and it is not surprising that some contradictory results occur. A substance given into a lateral cerebral ventricle or into the third ventricle can pass rapidly through the third ventricle and into the fourth ventricle, and may be spread over the ventral surface of the medulla and on to the surface of the spinal cord. On its way it is also in contact with the surface of the para-aqueductal grey matter. Thus it is potentially possible for the substance to enter brain tissue at many sites, and this may also depend on appropriate carrier systems at the csf–tissue interfaces. Should there be excitatory actions in one locus of penetration and inhibitory actions in others, then the resultant response may be the sum of the actions at several loci. It is hardly surprising then that, with so many variables in play, there are contradictory responses reported to the so-called 'central' action of compounds. The use of icv administration can be a useful starting-point in the investigation of a substance. But after this initial set of observations it is necessary to identify the tissue loci of action of substances and to use these as loci of administration of the test compound. Some other complicating technical problems often occur. Rarely is the pH of the material injected into brain tissue or cerebral ventricles described as being maintained precisely at the local tissue fluid or csf pH, and often there is little control of osmolality. Such apparently small control matters could, in some circumstances, have a major effect on responses. This cannot be ruled out by just injecting the vehicle as a control since the effect of the unusual pH or osmolality may only occur in the presence of the test material. Also, the techniques often used to render the fluid containers pyrogen free are thought to be adequately controlled by the responses to injections of vehicle handled in the same way, but minute amounts of endotoxin which of themselves have no effect could be additive to the effects of other substances added to the vehicle. The differences between the carefully planned experiments of Rothwell and of others will probably be resolved in terms of small differences in technique.

The action of CRF peripherally on fever caused by Poly I:Poly C has been studied by Milton *et al.* (1993a). They found that the usual bi-phasic fever caused by the pyrogen was blocked by anti-CRF antibodies or the CRF receptor antagonist, and this points to a peripheral role for CRF in this one type of fever. Also, Milton *et al.* (1992) have found activation of the hypothalamo-pituitary-adrenocortical axis in the rabbit by Poly I:Poly C; and they found evidence that this activation was CRF-41 dependent. The fever produced by the pyrogen and the rise in circulating PGE_2, as measured by radioimmunoassay, were blocked by a cyclo-oxygenase inhibitor, but the rise in serum cortisol was not and thus was probably not PGE dependent. They found evidence that the resting levels of cortisol in the absence of the pyrogen were both CRF-41 and PGE dependent. The pyrogen used is an interferon inducer and of course these results cannot be extrapolated to fevers induced by other cytokines.

While the part played by ACTH and peripheral antipyretic steroids could be an important part of the action of endogenous antipyretics there is much to be done to show that this is or is not the case. The evidence that AVP can reduce activity in glutamate excited neurons in the VSA is a good start for studies of this endogenous antipyretic. It still remains to be shown that such neurons are part of the fever mechanism, and the important projections from the septum used in antipyresis are virtually unknown. Whether there is a link between the action of AVP and

α-MSH is not known. The effects of AVP in adrenalectomized or hypophysectomized animals have not been studied. There remains the possibility that there are many endogenous antipyretics, not as evolutionary redundancies but as necessary units in a co-ordinated response to the multiplicity of infecting agents and cytokine mediators.

8

Febrile convulsions in children and a possible role for vasopressin

Fever and convulsions in infancy

A significant number of little children experience convulsive activity during episodes of infective and other fevers. Lorin (1982) suggests that 2–4% of all children have at least one fever-related seizure by the age of 5–7 years. Others (e.g. Miller *et al.*, 1960), have given a figure of 33/1000, or 3.3%, during the first five years of life. American studies tend to report a slightly higher incidence. While there is still some argument on the subject it seems likely that there is a genetic factor, a specific genetic trait transmitted by a low penetrance single dominant gene, in the predisposition to febrile convulsions in many cases (for review see Lennox-Buchtal, 1976). The distribution of the temperatures at which convulsions occur was studied by Herlitz (1941), and it was slightly skewed from a Gaussian distribution with a peak incidence at 39.5–40.5 °C. This distribution is shown in Fig. 8.1. Some children convulse in response to small increases in body temperature in mild infections and these seizures can be severe. There may be a relationship between the rate of body temperature rise and the development of seizures. There is little evidence concerning a possible mechanism for the triggering of febrile convulsions in children, and the animal models, which are few, do not include spontaneous convulsions in response to infectious fevers and are thus not entirely satisfactory.

There may be serious sequelae to febrile convulsions though, fortunately, most single or even double episodes have a benign long-term outcome. From figures given by Wallace (1976), of Edinburgh children examined within 6 to 24 hours after a febrile convulsion, 23% had normal neurological examination results, 26% had detectable hemiplegia, 20% had signs of cerebellar ataxia, and 6% had signs of upper motor neuron facial weakness with some in whom the signs were

127

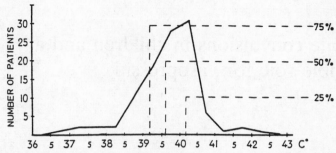

Fig. 8.1. Distribution of rectal temperatures at the time of a febrile convulsion or within 0.5 h in 104 babies. (From Herlitz, 1941.)

not clear. The author notes that on cursory routine examination the mild or minimal signs might not have been detected. The children in this study excluded those with known pre-existing neurological deficits. This study underlines the potential danger of febrile seizures and the need for very careful postictal neurological examination. The severe sequelae which may occur after prolonged or multiple convulsions include gross damage to neurological structures, impairment of mental development, the development of various types of epilepsy including temporal lobe epilepsy and behavioural disorders associated with damage to limbic structures (Lennox-Buchtal, 1976). The pre-existence of neurological abnormalities is of great importance in determining epilepsy as a sequela of febrile seizures, and may predispose to febrile convulsions. Much of the brain damage can be caused by anoxic ischaemia (Meldrum, 1976). The result can be sclerosis in the hippocampus and in some other brain areas. There may be pre-existing abnormalities which contribute also to the more severe neurological deficits seen after febrile seizures (Wallace, 1976). There may be a tendency in some cases to develop epileptic activity after episodes of febrile convulsions though this is still the subject of debate. The chances of occurrences of convulsive activity during fever, in the years in which febrile convulsions are most common, are increased following a first episode (Lorin, 1982). Phenobarbitone has been successfully used prophylactically in young severe cases, and diazepam may abort an episode, and of course reduction of the fever and treatment of its underlying cause are mandatory: lesions such as mesial temporal sclerosis may often be amenable to surgical treatment (Lennox-Buchtal, 1976).

Arginine vasopressin and seizure-like activity in rats

The extensive research in our laboratory on this topic started with an astute observation by Kasting (1980) who, during a study of the hypothermic action of arginine vasopressin given into the cerebral ventricles of the rat, noticed that the animal exhibited a brief period of staring, immobility and reduced respiration, and that a second dose of AVP evoked motor disturbances. Kruse *et al.* (1977) had previously described barrel rotations evoked by vasopressin and other peptides in rats. Wurpel *et al.* (1986) also described the occurrence of barrel rotation in rats in response to icv vasopressin. Kasting devised a behavioural score for the changes induced in which no effect was scored as '0'; brief staring, inaction and reduced respiration scored '1'; sprawling with extended hind limbs, mild ataxia and difficulty in walking scored '2'; overt motor disturbances including barrel rotation scored '3'; and full myoclonic seizures scored '4'. A dose of 1 μg AVP intraventricularly, in rats which had not previously had such treatment, gave a mean arithmetically averaged score of 1.5 on the above scale (Kasting *et al.*, 1980). The mean score in rats which received the same icv dose of AVP two days later was 3.5 with all showing barrel rotation or myoclonic seizures. On the fifth day after the first AVP injection a dose of 1.0 ng AVP given icv gave mean scores of 2.4. Saline controls had no motor disturbances. Thus it appeared that the first injection of AVP into a cerebral ventricle made the brain more sensitive to subsequent injections. Lederis *et al.* (1982) found that when rats were exposed to high environmental temperatures there was an excessive release of vasopressin in the brain and into the circulation and when the animals' temperatures reached 43 °C convulsions occurred. The threshold for convulsions was higher in rats which were passively immunized with vasopressin antiserum and in Brattleboro rats which are deficient in vasopressin. Burnard *et al.* (1983) were able to demonstrate an increase in motor disturbances evoked by icv vasopressin after administration of hypertonic saline intravenously or after haemorrhage, both of which treatments led to endogenous release of AVP in the rat brain. So not only can sensitization to the convulsive effects of AVP be induced by exogenously applied vasopressin, but also by endogenous release of the hormone.

Burnard *et al.* (1986) demonstrated that the AVP-V$_1$ receptor antagonist given icv in rats blocked both the motor disturbances in AVP

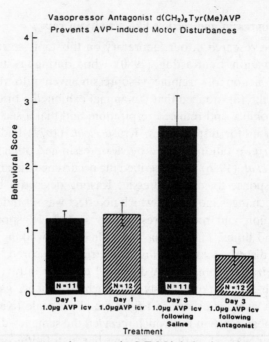

Fig. 8.2. Bars represent the mean (± S.E.M.) behavioural scores in response to 1.0 μg AVP icv. All rats receiving AVP on day 1 were given low behavioural scores, indicating a mild behavioural effect. On day 3, the control group (solid bars; n = 11) received 5.0 μl saline icv 5 min prior to AVP; the higher score indicates an increased severity of the motor disturbances observed. The group which received 1.0 μg antagonist (d(CH$_2$)$_5$Tyr(Me)AVP) icv 5 min prior to AVP on day 3 (slashed bars; n = 12) exhibited only minor behavioural anomalies, hence the antivasopressor analogue fully antagonized the severe motor disturbances normally observed following a second icv injection of AVP. (From Burnard *et al.*, 1986.)

sensitized animals (Fig. 8.2) and also blocked the sensitization process if administered immediately after the first icv dose of AVP. These authors also found evidence to suggest that the AVP-V$_2$ receptor was not involved.

Tissue injection of AVP has revealed one locus at which sensitization to the hormone causes severe motor disturbances in the rat (Naylor *et al.*, 1985; Naylor, 1987). AVP (100 ng) injected bilaterally into the ventral septal area produced on the first occasion a 12% incidence of convulsive behaviour, but a second challenge a day later caused an 88% incidence. Oxytocin (100 ng) bilaterally did not sensitize the brain to induce a high incidence of convulsions to a second dose of oxytocin (100 ng) a day later. Administration of the AVP-V$_1$ receptor antagonist into a lateral cerebral ventricle prevented the expected motor disturbances in rats given a second iv administration of AVP (Burnard *et al.*, 1986). These authors deduced, from the failure of a V_2 agonist to cause motor disturbances in rats previously primed with AVP, that the AVP-V_2 receptor is not involved in the sensitization process. Poulin & Pittman (1993a) found that oxytocin given icv sensitized the brain to produce severe motor disturbances when AVP was given by the same route 24 hours later in the rat. Thus, while the evidence supports the notion that the sensitization of the brain to motor disturbances may be mediated via the AVP-V_1 receptor, there may also be cross-sensitization by oxytocin via the oxytocin receptor. Synergistic interplay between the two receptors may occur. There is also evidence (Poulin & Pittman, 1993b) that the vasopressin-induced sensitization, which can be induced by AVP injections six hours to six days after a priming dose, may not involve alterations in AVP-V_1 receptor numbers, but may depend on post-receptor signal transduction mechanisms involving the hydrolysis of inositol phosphate. These authors found no changes in AVP-V_1 receptor density, as measured by [^{3}H]-AVP binding in the septal area neurons of sensitized animals. However, AVP stimulation of [^{3}H]-inositol monophosphate was clearly enhanced.

It has been known for some time (De Vries *et al.*, 1985) that there are vasopressin-containing terminals and vasopressin receptors (Dorsa *et al.*, 1984; Freund-Mercier *et al.*, 1988) in the amygdala in high concentrations. The increased vasopressin content of amygdala nerve terminals during fever has been demonstrated by Zeisberger *et al.* (1986). The amygdala is a locus in which kindling of convulsive activity can take place (Goddard, 1979). These considerations led Willcox *et al.* (1992) and Federico *et al.* (1992a) to investigate the amygdala as a possible site of sensitization to AVP in induction of AVP induced motor disturbances. Injection bilaterally of AVP (100 pmol in 1 μl sterile pyrogen free normal saline) on day 1 into the central medial amygdala caused minor motor responses such as immobility and mild ataxia and when this was followed by another identical injection 24 hours later there were severe motor responses which included barrel rotation and myoclonic seizures. Injections outside of the central medial amygdala, and control vehicle, did not induce marked motor responses. Prior administration into the amygdala locus of the AVP-V_1 receptor antagonist blocked the motor responses to both AVP injections. Thus it seems that the AVP dependent sensitization process in the amygdala is mediated via the AVP-V_1 receptors. Interestingly these authors also reported that administration of the AVP-V_2 receptor antagonist, while not blocking seizures in the sensitized animal, could sensitize the animal to further amygdala administration of AVP. This suggests that the process of sensitization may be brought about by multiple receptor systems. The amygdala can then be added to the septum as a region in which AVP can sensitize the brain in such a way that further release locally or administration locally of AVP can induce major motor disturbances. It is interesting that the loci at which AVP can engender motor disturbances coincide so well with the loci at which AVP exerts its endogenous antipyretic activity. This is good reason to explore further the possible role of AVP in febrile convulsions.

There is as yet no evidence that the AVP system is involved in the induction of febrile seizures in human children. Furthermore, the animal with an hereditary diathesis for febrile convulsions has not yet been found. However, the fact that there are extensive neuronal networks within the human brain which appear similar to those seen in the rat brain which are associated with the AVP responses, and that the rat can develop seizures associated with the neuronal networks involved in endogenous antipyresis, makes it worth while to pursue the (presently vague) possibility that the rat model described above could be of use in the study of human febrile convulsions. The endogenous antipyretic function of AVP is demonstrated in at least six species so far tested, but its presence in the human will await new non-invasive technologies for its substantiation. Such newly developing methodologies may well be able to test the hypothesis that the same system could be a part of the generation of febrile seizures in children.

9

A synthesis, predictions and speculations from my armchair

In 1798, James Currie wrote in his book *Medical Reports on the Effects of Water, Cold and Warm, as a Remedy in Fever and other Diseases* – 'The great difficulty which men have in all ages experienced in the acquisition of knowledge, has arisen from the promptitude of the human mind to decide in regard to causes. To the weak and ignorant, presumption is as natural as doubt is intolerable, and with such, belief is almost always a creature of the imagination. Nor is this peculiar to weakness and ignorance: to retain the mind unprejudiced and undecided in the investigation of striking and interesting phenomena, till by the painful steps of induction, the hidden cause is revealed, is an effort of the most difficult kind, and requires the highest and rarest powers of the understanding. The records of every part of science, bear ample testimony to this truth, particularly the records of medicine, and in a still more special manner that part of medicine which treats of the nature of fever. The most eminent physicians in every period of the world, impatient of observing and delineating, have been eager to explain and even to systematize; and the science of life owes its corruptions more to the misapplication of learning, than even to the dreams of superstition.' He then went on to say that the principles of the physical sciences and what could be termed engineering had been used to explain (or model) the functions of living things often with misleading results. So, in putting together a summary of some important aspects of our present knowledge about fever and antipyresis, I will try to indicate where there are gaps in our knowledge and what is hypothetical, and attempt not to systematize beyond the limits of the available evidence. I will also use some schematic diagrams which I hope will properly represent the current state of knowledge of the function of the nervous system in fever and antipyresis. In summarizing the present evidence, derived from

133

many sources, I will avoid re-quoting the references which are given fully in the preceding chapters.

Since the middle of this century there have been possibly five main advances in our understanding of the mechanisms of fever and antipyresis. First was the discovery of endogenous pyrogen and later the identification of several pyrogenic cytokines. Second came the association of prostaglandins with the mediation of the fever process and antipyresis. Third was the identification of loci of action of pyrogenic cytokines – circulating or released intracerebrally. Fourth has been the work showing the wide distribution of fever in the animal kingdom and the survival value of fever. Finally, was the elucidation of evidence supporting the notion of endogenous antipyretics, their loci of action, their action in modulating the extent of fever and their possible roles in suppressing fever in the peripartum.

The evidence already presented supports a widespread distribution in the animal kingdom of the ability to respond to infection with fever. It is, however, not ubiquitous, and sweeping conclusions cannot yet be safely made about the evolution and selection of the process of raising body temperature in response to infection as a useful individual survival strategy. Where it occurs there is good evidence for fever having a survival value, even in some mammals. However, it is important to bear in mind that there may also be a down side to fever. For example, in some cases, the occurrence of massive splanchnic area vasodilatation can tip the balance of survival in patients with compromised cardiac function.

In some species that get fever by behavioural means, i.e., by spending less time in the shade, this stratagem could lead to increased predation and elimination of the diseased individual from the rest of the group. This too is speculation. The ability to mount the other responses of the acute phase response without fever may be effective in some species, and much more needs to be done on the comparative immunology of infection and disease. I would suggest that neurophysiological studies on animals which have relatively simple nervous systems, made before and after challenge with pyrogens, could shed much light on the behavioural processes of fever, and possibly point the way for similar and useful studies in creatures having more complex nervous systems.

The evidence for the release of pyrogenic cytokines from tissue macrophages and monocytes in response to challenge with bacterial and viral products, which has grown out of the epoch-making discovery of endogenous pyrogen by Beeson (1948), is solid. However, it is now clear that there are several pyrogenic cytokines released and that the number of those discovered is still increasing. It is also clear that there are different cytokine pathways related to the different exogenous pyrogens or types of infection. It is then no longer valid to infer the whole process of all fevers from studies in which the responses to the iv or intracerebral administration of just one cytokine are used. That is not to say that valuable information, which might be common to the action of several other pyrogenic materials, cannot be gained by a detailed study of the action of a single pyrogen, but the temptation to extrapolate the results to apply to all fevers must be resisted.

To date the endogenous pyrogenic cytokines released in response to peripheral administration of bacterial and synthetic pyrogens, to bacterial infections and to viral challenges include IL-1$_\alpha$, IL-1$_\beta$, IL-6, TNF, IFN-α and IFN-β and MIP; and as this is being written I have little doubt that others are being found. The pyrogenic cytokines which have been studied in the greatest detail are the interleukins. The old notion that the pyrogenic cytokines in the systemic circulation diffuse to and have their primary action on the thermoregulatory structures within the hypothalamus is no longer tenable. The current wisdom is that they act at specialized regions of the brain where there are modifications of the blood–brain barrier, or within which are cells having receptors for the cytokines which can release further chemical messengers, or in which are neurons having cytokine receptors, the activation of which can provoke impulse traffic to the hypothalamic structures (Fig. 9.1). Of these regions receptive to the action of pyrogenic cytokines the evidence supports the circumventricular organs including the organum vasculosum of the lamina terminalis and possibly the area postrema as loci of action of IL-1. The subfornical organ does not appear to be involved, but a posterior hypothalamic/tuberal region might also be a site of pyrogen action and a midbrain reticular region has been suggested without very firm evidence. The OVLT appears also to be a locus of action of TNF and IFNs. Acting within the OVLT, pyrogenic cytokines have been shown to release PGE$_2$.

The next link is that from the special regions of action of the peripherally released pyrogenic cytokines to those parts of the thermoregulatory system responsible for increasing the body temperature and apparently raising the temperature set point. This is a much less complete part of the story. Pyrogenic cytokines can excite neurons within the OVLT, and there are projections from the OVLT to the AH/POA. There are IL-1-containing neurons within the AH/POA, and struc-

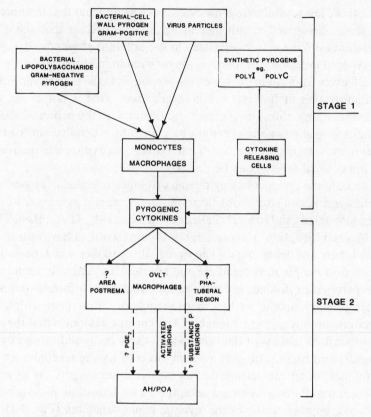

Fig. 9.1. The first stages of the fever mechanism (i.e., infection to the brain).

tures there can release PGE_2. It may be advantageous to have a cytokine/PGE_2 system within the hypothalamus, either as a secondary relay, the activation of which is evoked from pyrogens working on the circumventricular regions, or as a system which could respond to intracerebral infection or trauma. Whether the release of PGE_2 within the AH/POA is the sole mediation process of fever has been challenged and requires much more study. It is my present opinion that PGE_2 plays an important role particularly in the initial stage of fever, but that there are likely to be other pathways within the brain which can evoke fever without the participation of PGE_2. A suggestion has been that part of the link from the OVLT to the AH/POA may involve substance P-containing neurons. Another postulates excitation of OVLT neurons projecting to the AH/POA with subsequent excitation or inhibition of thermoresponsive neurons in the hypothalamic region. To date we have little information on the cytoarchitecture of the hypothalamic thermoregulatory apparatus or of the neurotransmitter sequences used there. Some valuable anatomical and neurophysiological information has been derived from hypothalamic slice studies, but the responses of neurons studied in this way are often of cells deprived of their usual afferent inputs, and their responses obviously cannot be correlated with the physiological thermoregulatory behaviour. There is evidence of actions of both prostaglandins and of pyrogenic cytokines on the behaviour of single thermosensitive neurons. This, as we have seen, is not completely consistent with the notion that these pyrogenic substances actually act via alterations in the hypothalamic thermosensitive structures; and this notion also faces the difficulty that the precise role of these structures in thermoregulation has not been clearly demonstrated in the awake-behaving animal. In the human the responses of the central warm receptors appear to be within the normal range during the plateau of fever but the core temperature behaves as though it is regulated about a new set level. There are many ideas as to how a new set level could be achieved including the alteration of the ionic constitution of the posterior hypothalamic interstitial fluid. None of these concepts has yet sufficient evidence for them to be strongly held hypotheses. It is also possible that the events emanating from the OVLT and the AH/POA in fever could result in a direct drive, not involving the usual thermoregulatory pathways, to the efferent neurons from the posterior hypothalamus with those neurons in a steady state of excitation still able to respond to stimuli from thermoregulatory circuits. Again, this is purely hypothetical.

A theoretical schema is given in Fig. 9.2. In this diagram, which is to a large extent hypothetical, I have attempted to put in circuitry which seems necessary for the afferent information and effector responses to bring about the rise in core temperature in fever. Some circuits will be of greater importance in certain species, e.g., those involving the NTS in non-shivering thermogenesis, or BAT, in the rat but which may not be of great importance in the human. We do not know the location of the set point apparatus, if it should exist, but I have placed it between the AH/POA and the posterior hypothalamus in the diagram, but it might be located in either or both. I have made the posterior hypothalamus into a final common path for the efferent systems for fever and this may be an over-simplification. The shivering mechanism is shown in the figure to involve both the hypothalamic nuclei and the septal area and there is some good evidence for this. It also seems

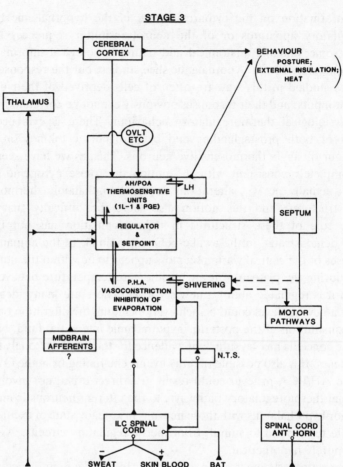

Fig. 9.2. The possible pathways involved between the arrival of pyrogenic cytokines at the brain and the efferent mechanisms causing fever.

probable that afferents from the cold receptors in the skin, which would be cooled as the skin circulation is greatly reduced in fever, can contribute to the intensity and possibly to the initiation of shivering. The locus of origin of the neurons which initiate shivering during fever is unknown, but if there is a system to raise the temperature set point then they must be connected with it. It could be, as I have tentatively suggested earlier, that the drive originating in some circumventricular organs and mediated via the AH/POA could be outside the normally used thermoregulatory apparatus, and could directly drive the heat production and heat conservation systems at some final common path locus.

Afferent information from the cold receptors in the skin is likely to travel by the usual spinal pathways and thalamic relays to connect with the hypothalamic regions, and also to relay to the sensorimotor cortex for the conscious experience of intense cold and for initiation of behavioural responses for body warming.

Efferents from hypothalamic regions travel via pathways involving medullary vasomotor control regions to the intermediolateral columns of the spinal cord. There they relay to the preganglionic sympathetic neurons to connect with α-adrenergic postganglionic fibres distributed to skin blood vessels. The cholinergic sympathetic neurons innervating sweat glands are inhibited during the rising temperature phase of fever, and excited during the defervescence phase. Other neurons relay in the nucleus of the tractus solitarius to connect with efferent neurons going to the intermediolateral column of the spinal cord with further relays to β-adrenergic fibres to BAT regions in appropriate species.

The problem still remains to identify and locate the central mechanism(s) which regulate the process of fever. I have touched on this problem already in this chapter, but the matter deserves some further consideration. Is there a neural process which sets the normal core temperature and raises that set point during fever? Evidence from human and other experiments supports the notion that the thermoregulatory system behaves as though this were the case. Schemata involving the response of warm and cold responsive neurons in the hypothalamic/septal areas to pyrogenic cytokines and prostaglandins have been drawn up with the suggestion that the pyrogens inhibit warm receptor activity and enhance that of cold receptors. The evidence concerning this is far from convincing. An alternative hypothesis is that the pyrogenic final mediators act on pathways not usually used in thermoregulation to evoke heat production and conservation responses and inhibit the heat loss responses. At the plateau of fever the response to central and peripheral thermoreceptor stimulation evokes normal thermoregulatory behaviours. This notion requires that the firing range of 'central' thermoreceptors is linear, or close to linear, and extends over a very wide range of temperature. There is some evidence (see Chapter 6) that reflex vasodilatation in the hand in response to body trunk exposure to radiant heat, which is inhibited in fever, can be demonstrated by overcoming the fever-induced skin vasoconstriction by local heating. In other words, the stimulation of the skin warm receptive mechanism and the induced reflex is operational but masked by high vasoconstrictor tone during fever. While there is evidence for there being a wide range of temperature over which thermoreceptors, both central (Cooper, 1970) and peripheral, can operate, the hypothesis suggested above which does not involve an alteration in a temperature set point is also far from convincing. Until we have a much better understanding of the hypothalamic-septal-brainstem cytoarchitecture of thermoregulatory pathways and of the integrative thermoregulatory mechanisms we cannot answer the fundamental questions about the way in which pyrogenic mediators cause fever. To use Currie's words, it is our great temptation to 'explain and even to systematize' before we have adequate data. While it may be to some extent true that often the teaching of science is a process of diminishing deception, the dogmatic statements about the nature of fever, which appear in many textbooks, cater mainly to the discomfort which the mediocre student has with doubt, rather than to the stimulation of the student's critical abilities! The diagrams used in this chapter serve only as pegs on which to hang the discussions and it is my earnest hope that they will not be copied into textbooks as true records of the fever and antipyresis processes.

A final diagram, Fig. 9.3, outlines our present ideas of endogenous antipyretic systems within the brain, and again the concept shown here is far from complete and will probably require much modification before long. It shows the presently known pathways for two peptides which appear to act to limit the extent of fever. The one, AVP, involves neurons originating in the paraventricular nucleus and the bed nucleus of the stria terminalis which project to the ventral septal area in the vicinity of the diagonal band of Broca. Stimulation of release of AVP from these neurons, or local micro-injection of AVP, reduces fever caused by iv injection of bacterial pyrogen, pyrogenic cytokines and intraventricular administration of pyrogenic cytokines and prostaglandins by an AVP-V_1 receptor mediated mechanism. The medial amygdaloid nucleus also seems to be a locus of action of AVP as an antipyretic. The recent evidence for induction of septal release of AVP by action of IL-1 on the BST is an important possible addition to our knowledge of the mechanism of AVP release during fever.

The other endogenous antipyretic system involves the release of α-MSH into the lateral septum from neurons originating in the arcuate nucleus, and of some release of α-MSH into the peripheral circulation where it has antipyretic and anti-inflammatory actions. There is also

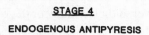

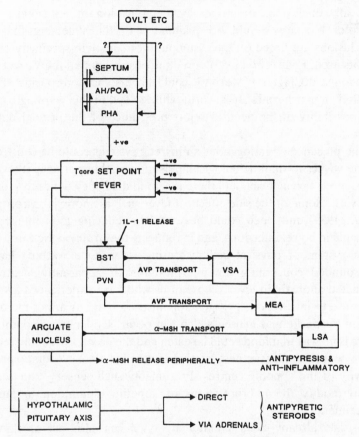

Fig. 9.3. Possible pathways involved in endogenous antipyresis.

evidence for stimulation of the hypothalamic/pituitary axis to cause, directly or indirectly, release of antipyretic steroids.

A good deal of the arguments relating to the actions of cytokines, fever mediators and endogenous antipyretics within the brain is dependent on the alteration in their responses by receptor blocking agents and substance antagonists. This is probably reasonable, but there always remains one obstacle. The local application of the compounds is done on the assumption that they have specific and only one action. One is reminded of the problem of local intracerebral administration of propranolol in studying monoamine action, and the problem which arose when it was discovered that at many of the concentrations at which it was used propranolol could act as a local anaesthetic. It seems to me that all conclusions based on local application of antagonists and receptor blockers should be qualified with the statement that the conclusions are based on the assumption of complete specificity of the agents used. Fyda *et al.* (1989) raised the possibility that the V_1 receptor antagonist $d(CH_3)_5Try(Me)AVP$ could have some non-specific effects on PGE hyperthermia. It is worth while to sound this warning even if the possibility of the need to reinterpret much of the present data is remote.

The presence of endogenous antipyretic systems could be construed, if one wishes to think teleologically, as of special importance if fever is considered as beneficial, and there is a good deal of evidence to support this view. Some of the side effects of fever such as anorexia (Mrosovsky *et al.*, 1989) and sleep could be useful in reducing food intake, for example in bowel infections, and in reducing the strain on the cardiovascular system of physical activity during fever. One warning has to be sounded concerning the interpretation of apparently 'centrally' mediated anorexia in fever. Those of us who have experienced fever in response to intravenous pyrogen administration are aware of the often severe headache and nausea which can occur. Under these conditions there is no way that food could be eaten and the process probably relates more to the unpleasantness of the experience than to some specific activity of the appetite centres. Presumably such sensory experiences could modify the interpretations of appetite diminution in animal experiments.

As has already been mentioned, AVP can also act to 'kindle' seizure-like activity (or severe motor disturbances) and this should not only be considered as a possibly disadvantageous side effect but should stimulate research into a possible causal relationship between AVP release and febrile convulsions in children. To date such a relationship is purely hypothetical but deserves investigation. A possible role of AVP acting within the brain in the genesis of tolerance to endotoxin requires a good deal more investigation. Is it one of many causes of tolerance or does it play a critical role? Certainly the high mortality of young animals made tolerant to bacterial pyrogen and given indomethacin, and the role of AVP in this, needs more study as a possible model of Reye's syndrome.

Despite some of the possible deleterious side effects of AVP release, and this release may be part of the action of some antipyretic drugs, and with the evidence for a survival value of fever, I would not advise withholding of temperature-lowering procedures in severe fevers. It is likely, based on a few mammalian studies, that the advantages gained from fever are complete by the time the patient consults a physician, i.e., 6–12 hours from the onset of symptoms.

In all that has been discussed relating to both the functions of the CNS in fever and antipyresis there seems to be an emerging concept of involvement of many more brain regions than just the hypothalamus in their initiation and maintenance, apart from the multiple efferent pathways. The use of new and more precise technologies will confirm or refute such ideas and enable us to define the circuitry more clearly. It is difficult to predict which research projects are most likely to be fruitful in the future. Prediction is likely to be rendered inaccurate by two factors, namely, the development of new technologies and serendipity, and these cannot be foretold. But, the development of methods for studying the relationship between neuronal activity and thermoregulatory behaviour, and of visualizing active brain regions, ethically, in conscious and unrestrained animals seems to hold out much promise. The only prediction which is safe is that the way to advance our knowledge of fever and its mechanisms is in the words of T. H. Huxley (1860), 'Sit down before fact as a little child, be prepared to give up every preconceived notion, follow humbly wherever and to whatever abysses nature leads, or you shall learn nothing.'

Those coming into the field of research, into the role of the nervous system in fever and antipyresis have much to accomplish and the promise of a great intellectual adventure.

Appendix 1. Anatomical considerations

This short appendix consists of a few anatomical diagrams to supplement those in the main text. For detailed diagrams of neuronal pathways using monoaminergic, peptidergic, cholinergic and substance P containing neurons the reader is referred to Nieuwenhuys *Chemoarchitecture of the Brain* (1985), Springer-Verlag, Berlin; New York.

The diagrams printed in this appendix include a whole brain sagittal section to show the location of the third ventricle; another such section

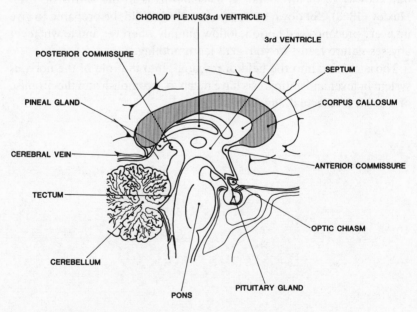

Fig. A1.1. Sagittal brain section through the third ventricle.

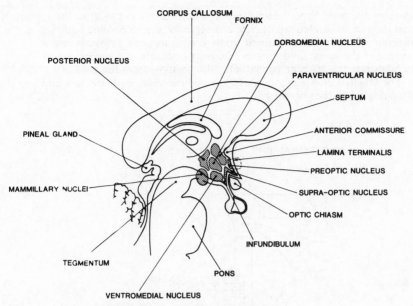

Fig. A1.2. Sagittal brain section showing hypothalamic nuclei.

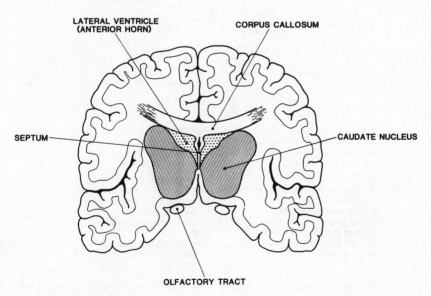

Fig. A1.3. Coronal brain section through the anterior horns of the lateral ventricles.

showing the main hypothalamic nuclei; a coronal section to show the septum and the lateral cerebral ventricles; a diagram of the autonomic outflows; a diagram of the intracerebral and spinal cord autonomic pathways and a section of the spinal cord to show the intermediolateral columns and to demonstrate the efferent sympathetic fibre outflow from the cord.

The labelled drawings are intended to be complete in themselves and requiring no further comment.

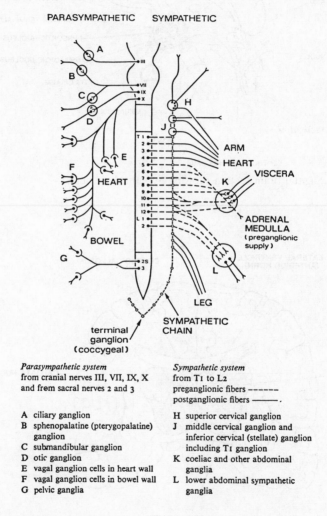

Parasympathetic system	Sympathetic system
from cranial nerves III, VII, IX, X	from T1 to L2
and from sacral nerves 2 and 3	preganglionic fibers ------
	postganglionic fibers ———.

A ciliary ganglion	H superior cervical ganglion
B sphenopalatine (pterygopalatine) ganglion	J middle cervical ganglion and inferior cervical (stellate) ganglion including T1 ganglion
C submandibular ganglion	
D otic ganglion	K coeliac and other abdominal ganglia
E vagal ganglion cells in heart wall	
F vagal ganglion cells in bowel wall	L lower abdominal sympathetic ganglia
G pelvic ganglia	

Fig. A1.4. The peripheral autonomic nervous system. (From Johnson & Spalding, 1974.)

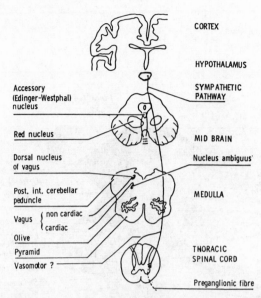

Fig. A1.5. On the right the course of sympathetic pathways from the hypothalamus to the cells in the intermediolateral columns of the thoracic spinal cord, from which arise the preganglionic sympathetic fibres. On the left the origin of parasympathetic fibres in the third and tenth cranial nerves. (From Johnson & Spalding, 1974.)

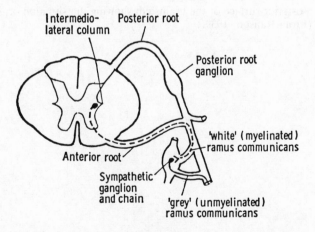

Fig. A1.6. Relationship of preganglionic (---) and postganglionic (——) sympathetic fibres with nerve roots and sympathetic chain. (From Johnson & Spalding, 1974.)

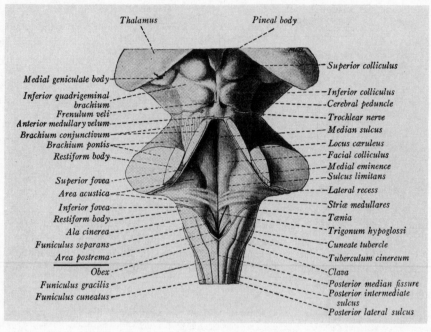

Fig. A1.7. Posterior surface of the brainstem showing the situation of the area postrema. (From Ranson, 1939.)

References

There are a number of papers listed that are not mentioned within the text, it was felt that these were of sufficient importance that they should be included for completeness.

Abscher, M. & Stineberg, W. R. (1969). Toxic properties of a synthetic double stranded RNA. Endotoxin like properties of Poly I;Poly C, an interferon stimulator. *Nature*, **223**, 715–17.

Alexander, D. P., Bashore, R. A., Britton, R. A. & Forsling, M. A. (1974). Maternal and fetal arginine vasopressin in the chronically catheterized sheep. *Biol. Neonate.*, **25**, 242–8.

Alexander, S. J., Cooper, K. E. & Veale, W. L. (1989). Sodium salicylate: alternate mechanism of central antipyretic action in the rat. *Pflügers Arch.*, **413**, 451–5.

Allen, I. V. (1965). The cerebral effects of endogenous serum and granulocytic pyrogen. *Brit. J. Exptl. Path.*, **46**, 25–34.

Amin, A. N., Crawford, T. B. B. & Gaddum, J. H. (1954). The distribution of substance P and 5-hydroxytryptamine in the central nervous system of the dog. *J. Physiol. (Lond)*, **126**, 596–618.

Andersson, B. (1957). Cold defense reactions elicited by electrical stimulation within the septal area of the brain in goats. *Acta Physiol. Scand.*, **41** (Fasc.1), 90–100.

Andersson, B. & Larsson, B. (1961). Influence of local temperature changes in the preoptic area and rostral hypothalamus on the regulation of food and water intake. *Acta. Physiol. Scand.*, **52**, 75–89.

Appenzeller, O. & Schnieden, H. (1963). Neurogenic pathways concerned in reflex vasodilatation in the hand, with special reference to stimuli affecting the afferent pathway. *Clin. Sci.*, **25**, 413–21.

Atkins, E. & Snell, E. S. (1964). A comparison of the biological properties of Gram-negative bacterial endotoxin with leucocyte and tissue pyrogens. In *Bacterial Endotoxins*, ed. M. Landy & W. Braun, pp. 134–48. Rutgers Univ. Press, New Brunswick.

Auron, P. E., Webb, A. C., Rosenwasser, L. J., Mucci, S. F., Rich, A., Wolff, S. M. & Dinarello, C. A. (1984). Nucleotide sequence of human monocyte interleukin-1 precursor cDNA. *Proc. Natl. Acad. Sci. USA*, **81**, 7909–11.

Banet, M. & Wieland, U.-E. (1985). The effect of intraseptally applied vasopressin on thermoregulation in the rat. *Brain Res. Bull.*, **14**, 113–16.

Banks, W. A., Kastin, A. J. & Durham, D. A. (1989). Bidirectional transport of interleukin-1 alpha across the blood brain barrier. *Brain Res. Bull.*, **23**, 43–7.

Bannister, R. G. (1960). Anhidrosis following intravenous pyrogen. *Lancet*, **ii**, 118–22.

Barker, J. L. & Carpenter, D. O. (1970). Thermosensitivity of neurons in the sensorimotor cortex of the cat. *Science*, **169**, 597–8.

Bazett, H. C. & McGlone, B. (1930). Experiments on the mechanism of stimulation of end-organs for cold. *Amer. J. Physiol.*, **93**, 632.

Beeson, P. B. (1947). Tolerance to bacterial pyrogens. II. Role of the reticuloendothelial system. *J. Expt. Med.*, **86**, 39–44.

Beeson, P. B. (1948). Temperature-elevating effect of a substance obtained from polymorphonuclear leucocytes. *J. Clin. Invest.*, **27**, 524.

Bell, R. C. & Lipton, J. M. (1987). Pulsatile release of antipyretic neuropeptide α-MSH from septum of rabbit during fever. *Amer. J. Physiol.*, **252**, R1152–7.

Bennet, I. L. & Beeson, P. B. (1953a). Studies on the pathogenesis of fever. I. The effect of injection of extracts and suspensions of uninfected rabbit tissues upon the body temperature of normal rabbits. *J. Exptl. Med.*, **98**, 477–92.

Bennet, I. L. & Beeson, P. B. (1953b). Studies in the pathogenesis of fever. II. Characterization of fever-producing substances from polymorphonuclear leukocytes and from the fluid of sterile exudates. *J. Exp. Med.*, **98**, 493–508.

Benzinger, T. H. & Taylor, G. W. (1963). Cranial measurements of internal temperature in man. In *Temperature: Its Measurement and Control in Science and Industry*, vol.3. pt.3, ed. J. D. Hardy (pp. 637–65). Reinhold, New York.

Bernadini, G. L., Lipton, J. M. & Clark, W. G. (1983). Intracerebroventricular and septal injections of arginine vasopressin are not antipyretic in the rabbit. *Peptides*, **4**, 195–8.

Bernadini, G. L., Richards, D. B. & Lipton, J. M. (1984). Antipyretic effect of centrally administered CRF. *Peptides*, **5**, 57–9.

Bernheim, H. A. & Kluger, M. J. (1976a). Fever and antipyresis in the lizard Dipsosaurus dorsalis. *Amer. J. Physiol.*, **231**, 198–203.

Bernheim, H. A. & Kluger, M. J. (1976b). Fever: effect of drug-induced antipyresis on survival. *Science*, **193**, 237–9.

Bernheim, H. A. & Kluger, M. J. (1977). Endogenous pyrogen-like substance produced by reptiles. *J. Physiol. (Lond)*, **267**, 659–66.

Bertler, Å. (1961). Occurrence and localization of catechol amines in the human brain. *Acta Physiol. Scand.*, **51**, 97–107.

Bidstrup, P. L. & Payne, D. J. H. (1951). Poisoning by dinitro-ortho-cresol. Report of eight fatal cases occurring in Great Britain. *Brit. Med. J.*, **2**, (July), 1–11.

Bito, L. Z. & Davson, H. (1974). Carrier-mediated removal of prostaglandins from cerebrospinal fluid. *J. Physiol. (Lond)*, **236**, 39–40P.

Blatteis, C. M. (1990a). Neuromodulative actions of cytokines. *The Yale J. Biol. Med.*, **63**, 133–46.

Blatteis, C. M. (1990b). The neurobiology of endogenous pyrogen. In *Thermoreception and Temperature Regulation*, ed. J. Bligh & K. Voigt, pp. 257–72. Springer-Verlag, Berlin.

Blatteis, C. M. (1992). The OVLT: the interface between the brain and circulating pyrogens? In *Neuro-immunology of Fever*, ed. T. Bartfai & D. Ottoson, pp. 167–76. Pergamon Press, Oxford.

Blatteis, C. M. & Banet, M. (1986). Autonomic thermoregulation after separation of the preoptic area from the hypothalamus in rats. *Pflügers Arch.*, **406**, 480–4.

Blatteis, C. M., Bealer, S. L., Hunter, W. A., Llanos-Q, J., Ahokas, R. A. & Mashburn, T. A. (1983a). Suppression of fever after lesions of the anteroventral third ventricle in guinea pigs. *Brain Res. Bull.*, **11**, 519–26.

Blatteis, C. M., Hunter, W. S., Llanos, J., Ahokas, R. A. & Mashburn, T. A. (1983b). The preoptic area (PO) mediates the acute phase response (APR) in guinea pigs. *Fed. Proc.*, **42** (464), Abst. 1008.

Blatteis, C. M., Hales, J. R. S., McKinley, M. J. & Fawcett, A. A. (1987). Role of the anteroventral third ventricle in fever in sheep. *Can. J. Physiol. Pharm.*, **65**, 1255–60.

Blatteis, C. M., Hales, J. R. S., Fawcett, A. A. & Mashburn, T. A. (1988). Fever and regional blood flow in wethers and parturient sheep. *J. Appl. Physiol.*, **65**, 165–72.

Bligh, J. (1972). Neuronal models of mammalian temperature regulation. In *Essays on Temperature Regulation*, ed. J. Bligh & R. E. Moore, pp. 105–20. North Holland, Amsterdam.

Bligh, J. (1973). *Temperature Regulation in Mammals and other Vertebrates*. North-Holland, Amsterdam.

Bligh, J., Silver, A. & Smith, C. A. (1977). A central cholinergic synapse between cold sensors and heat production effectors in the sheep: True or false? *J. Physiol. (Lond)*, **266**, 88–9P.

Bodel, P. & Atkins, E. (1967). Release of endogenous pyrogen by human monocytes. *N. Eng. J. Med.*, **276**, 1002–8.

Boorstein, S. M. & Ewald, P. W. (1987). Costs and benefits of behavioral fever in *Melanoplus sanguinipes* infected by *Nosema acridophagus*. *Physiol. Zool.*, **60**, 586–95.

Borsook, D., Laburn, H. & Mitchell, D. (1978). The febrile responses in rabbits and rats to leucocyte pyrogens of different species. *J. Physiol. (Lond)*, **279**, 113–20.

Boulant, J. A. & Dean, J. B. (1987). Reception and integration of thermal information in horizontal hypothalamic tissue slices. In *Selected Topics in Hypothalamic Research*. Proc. of Satellite Symposium to the Second World Congress of Neurosciences (August 12–14), p. 34. Budapest, Hungary.

Boulant, J. A., Curras, M. C. & Dean, J. B. (1989). Neurophysiological Aspects of Thermoregulation. In *Advances in Comparative and Environmental Physiology*, vol.4, ed. L. C. H. Wang, pp. 117–60. Springer-Verlag, Berlin.

Bradley, S. E. & Conan, N. J. (1947). Estimated hepatic blood flow and bromosulfophthalein extraction in normal man during pyrogenic reaction. *J. Clin. Invest.*, **26**, 1175.

Braude, A. I., Zalesky, M. & Douglas, H. (1958). The mechanism of tolerance to fever. *J. Clin. Invest.*, **37**, 880–1.

Braude, A. L., McConnell, J. & Douglas, H. (1960). Fever from pathogenic fungi. *J. Clin. Invest.*, **39**, 1266–76.

Breder, C. D. & Saper, C. B. (1988). Tumor necrosis factor immunoreactive innervation in the mouse brain. *Soc. Neurosci.*, Abst. 14, 1280.

Breder, C. D., Dinarello, C. A. & Saper, C. B. (1988). Interleukin-1 immunoreactive innervation of the human hypothalamus. *Science*, **240**, 321–3.

Breder, C. D., Smith, W. L., Raz, A., Masferrer, J., Siebert, K., Needleman, P. & Saper, C. B. (1992). Distribution and characterization of cyclooxygenase immunoreactivity in the ovine brain. *J. Comp. Neurol.*, **322**, 409–38.

Brodie, B. B. & Shore, P. A. (1957). A concept for a role of serotonin and norepinephrine as chemical mediators in the brain. *Ann. N. Y. Acad. Sci.*, **66**, 631–42.

Bronstein, S. M. & Conner, W. E. (1984). Endotoxin induced behavioural fever in the Madagascar cockroach Gramphadorhina portentosa. *J. Insect Physiol.*, **30**, 327–30.

Brück, K. (1961). Temperature regulation in the newborn infant. *Biol. Neonat. (Basel)*, **3**, 65–119.

Brück, K. (1978). Heat production and temperature regulation. In *Perinatal Physiology*, ed. U. Stave, pp. 455–98. Plenum Publishing Co., N. York.

Brück, K. & Hinckel, P. (1980). Thermoregulatory noradrenergic and serotonergic pathways to hypothalamic units. *J. Physiol. (Lond)*, **304**, 193–202.

Bryce-Smith, R., Coles, D. R., Cooper, K. E., Cranston, W. I. & Goodale, F. (1959). The effects of intravenous pyrogen upon the radiant heat induced vasodilatation in man. *J. Physiol. (Lond)*, **145**, 77–84.

Buijs, R. M., Swaab, D. F., Dogterom, J. & van Leewen, F. W. (1978). Intra- and extrahypothalamic vasopressin and oxytocin pathways in the rat. *Cell Tiss. Res.*, **186**, 423–33.

Burnard, D. M., Pittman, Q. J. & Veale, W. L. (1983). Increased motor disturbances in response to arginine vasopressin following hemorrhage and hypertonic saline: evidence for AVP release in rats. *Brain. Res.*, **273**, 59–65.

Burnard, D. M., Veale, W. L. & Pittman, Q. J. (1986). Prevention of arginine- vasopressin-induced motor disturbances by a potent vasopressor antagonist. *Brain Res.*, **362**, 40–6.

Cabanac, M. & LeGuelte, L. (1980). Temperature regulation and prostaglandin E_1 fever in scorpions. *J. Physiol. (Lond)*, **303**, 365–70.

Cabanac, M. & Rossetti, Y. (1987). Fever in snails, reflections on a negative result. *Comp. Biochem. Physiol.*, **87**A, 1017–20.

Cabanac, M., Chatonnet, J. & Philipot, R. (1965). Les conditions de témpératurés cérébrale et cutanée moyennes pour l'apparition du frisson thermique chez le chien. *C. R. Acad. Sci. (Paris)*, **260**, 680–3.

Cabanac, M., Stolwijk, J. A. & Hardy, J. D. (1968). Effect of temperature and pyrogens on single unit activity in the rabbit's brain stem. *J. Appl. Physiol.*, **24**, 645–52.

Cannon, J. G., Granowitz, E. V., Dinarello, C. A. & Wolff, S. M. (1992). Responses of humans to bacterial endotoxin. In *Neuro-Immunology of Fever*, ed. T. Bartfai & D. Ottoson, pp. 97–106. Pergamon Press, Oxford.

Carlsson, A., Falck, B., Hillarp, N. & Torp, A. (1962). Histochemical localization at the cellular level of hypothalamic noradrenaline. *Acta Physiol. Scand.*, **54**, 385–6.

Casterlin, M. E. & Reynolds, W. W. (1977). Behavioral fever in anuran amphibian larvae. *Life Sci.*, **20**, 593–6.

Casterlin, M. E. & Reynolds, W. W. (1978). Prostaglandin E_1 fever in the crayfish *Cambarus bartoni*. *Pharmacol. Biochem. Behav.*, **9**, 593–5.

Cechetto, D. F. & Saper, C. B. (1990). Role of the cerebral cortex in autonomic function. In *Central Regulation of Autonomic Functions*, ed. A. D. Loewy & K. M. Spyer, pp. 208–23. Oxford University Press, Oxford.

Chambers, W. W., Koenig, H., Koenig, R. & Windle, W. F. (1949). Site of action in the central nervous system of bacterial pyrogen. *Amer. J. Physiol.*, **159**, 209–16.

Chassis, H., Ranges, H. A., Goldring, W. & Smith, H. W. (1938). The control of renal blood flow and glomerular filtration in normal man. *J. Clin. Invest.*, **17**, 683–97.

Clark, W. G. (1991). Antipyretics. In *Fever: Basic Mechanisms and Management*, ed. P. Mackowiak, pp. 297–340. Raven Press Ltd., New York.

Coceani, F. (1991). Prostaglandins and fever – facts and controversies. In *Fever: Basic Mechanisms and Management*, ed. P. Mackowiak, pp. 59–70. Raven Press Ltd., New York.

Coceani, F. & Wolfe, L. S. (1966). On the actions of prostaglandin E_1 and prostaglandins from brain on the isolated rat stomach. *Can. J. Physiol. Pharmacol.*, **44**, 933–50.

Collins, K. J., Dore, C., Exton-Smith, A. N., Fox, R. H., MacDonald, I. C. & Woodward, P. M. (1977). Accidental hypothermia and impaired temperature homeostasis in the elderly. *Brit. Med. J.*, 1, 353–6.

Cooper, K. E. (1965a). Quantitative observations in disordered temperature regulation. In *The Scientific Basis of Medicine Annual Reviews*, p. 250. Athlone Press, London.

Cooper, K. E. (1965b). The role of the hypothalamus in the generation of fever. *Proc. R. Soc. Med.*, **58**, 740.

Cooper, K. E. (1970). Studies of the human central warm receptor. In *Physiological and Behavioral Temperature Regulation*, ed. J. D. Hardy, A. P. Gagge & J. A. L. Stolwijk, pp. 224–30. Charles C. Thomas, Publisher. Springfield, Ill., USA.

Cooper, K. E. (1987). The neurobiology of fever: thoughts on recent developments. *Ann. Rev. of Neurosci.*, **10**, 297–324.

Cooper, K. E. & Cranston, W. I. (1963). Clearance of radioactive bacterial pyrogen from the circulation. *J. Physiol. (Lond)*, **166**, 41–2P.

Cooper, K. E. & Cranston, W. I. (1966). Pyrogens and monoamine oxidase inhibitors. *Nature*, **210**, 203–4.

Cooper, K. E. & Kenyon, J. R. (1957). A Comparison of Temperatures measured in the Rectum, Oesophagus and on the surface of the Aorta during Hypothermia in Man. *Brit. J. Surg.*, **44**, 616–19.

Cooper, K. E. & Kerslake, D. McK. (1953). Abolition of nervous reflex vasodilatation by sympathectomy of the heated area. *J. Physiol. (Lond)*, **119**, 18–29.

Cooper, K. E. & Kerslake, D. McK. (1954). Some aspects of the reflex control of the cutaneous circulation. In *Peripheral Circulation in Man*, ed. G. E. W. Wolstenholme & J. S. Freeman, pp. 143–9. J. & A. Churchill Ltd, London.

Cooper, K. E. & Veale, W. L. (1972). The effect of an inert oil in the cerebral ventricular system upon fever produced by intravenous pyrogen. *Can. J. Physiol. Pharmacol.*, **50**, 1066–71.

Cooper, K. E. & Veale, W. L. (1994). Emerging themes in thermoregulation and fever. In *Temperature Regulation, Recent Physiological and Pharmacological Advances*, ed. A. S. Milton, pp. 357–67. Birkhäuser Verlag, Basel.

Cooper, K. E., Ferres, H. & Guttman, L. (1957). Vasomotor responses in the foot to raising body temperature in the paraplegic patient. *J. Physiol. (Lond)*, **136**, 547–55.

Cooper, K. E., Cranston, W. I., Dempster, W. J. & Mottram, R. F. (1960). Pyrogen-induced vasodilatation in the transplanted kidney. *J. Physiol. (Lond)*, **155**, 21–2P.

Cooper, K. E., Johnson, R. H. & Spalding, J. M. K. (1964a). Thermoregulatory reactions following intravenous pyrogen in a subject with complete transection of the cervical cord. *J. Physiol. (Lond)*, **171**, 55–6P.

Cooper, K. E., Johnson, R. H. & Spalding, J. M. K. (1964b). The effects of central body and trunk skin temperatures on reflex vasodilatation in the hand. *J. Physiol. (Lond)*, **174**, 46–54.

Cooper, K. E., Cranston, W. I. & Snell, E. S. (1964c). Temperature regulation during fever in man. *Clin. Sci.*, **27**, 345–56.

Cooper, K. E., Cranston, W. I. & Snell, E. S. (1964d). Temperature in the External Auditory Meatus as an index of central temperature changes. *J. Appl. Physiol.*, **19**, 1032–5.

Cooper, K. E., Cranston, W. I. & Honour, A. J. (1965). Effects of intraventricular and intra-hypothalamic injection of noradrenaline and 5-HT on body temperature in conscious rabbits. *J. Physiol. (Lond)*, **181**, 852–64.

Cooper, K. E., Cranston, W. I. & Honour, A. J. (1966). The site of action of leucocyte pyrogen in the rabbit brain. *J. Physiol. (Lond)*, **186**, 22P.

Cooper, K. E., Cranston, W. I. & Honour, A. J. (1967). Observations on the site and mode of action of pyrogens in the rabbit brain. *J. Physiol. (Lond)*, **191**, 325–37.

Cooper, K. E., Preston, E. & Veale, W. L. (1976). Effects of atropine injected into a lateral cerebral ventricle of the rabbit, on fevers due to intravenous leucocyte pyrogen and hypothalamic and intraventricular injections of prostaglandin E_1. *J. Physiol. (Lond)*, **254**, 729–41.

Cooper, K. E., Kasting, N. W., Lederis, K. & Veale, W. L. (1979). Evidence supporting a role for endogenous vasopressin in natural suppression of fever in the sheep. *J. Physiol. (Lond)*, **295**, 33–45.

Cooper, K. E., Naylor, A. M. & Veale, W. L. (1987). Evidence supporting a role for endogenous vasopressin in fever suppression in the rat. *J. Physiol. (Lond)*, **387**, 163–72.

Cooper, K. E., Blähser, S., Malkinson, T. J., Merker, G., Roth, J. & Zeisberger, E. (1988). Changes in body temperature and vasopressin content of brain neurons, in pregnant and non-pregnant guinea pigs, during fevers produced by Poly I:Poly C. *Pflügers Arch.*, **412**, 292–6.

Cooper, K. E., Malkinson, T. J., Monda, M., Pittman, Q. J. & Veale, W. L. (1992). New neurobiological concepts of the genesis of fever and of antipyresis. In *Neuro-immunology of Fever*, ed. T. Bartfai & D. Otoson, pp. 225–34. Pergamon Press, Oxford.

Cox, B. & Lee, T. F. (1982). Role of central neurotransmitters in fever. In *Pyretics and Antipyretics*, ed. A. S. Milton, pp. 125–50. Springer-Verlag, Berlin.

Cranston, W. I. (1959a). Experimental observations on human fever. *Ned. T. Geneesk.*, **103** (I), 5–8. Genootschap ter bevordering van natuur-genees-en heelkunde te Amsterdam. Symposium, May 11. 1957.

Cranston, W. I. (1959b). Fever, pathogenesis and circulatory changes. *Circulation*, **20**, 1133–42.

Cranston, W. I. (1979). Central mechanisms of fever. *Fed. Proc.*, **38**, 49–51.

Cranston, W. I., Gerbrandy, J. & Snell, E. S. (1954). Oral, Rectal and oesophageal Temperatures and some factors affecting them in Man. *J. Physiol. (Lond)*, **126**, 347–58.

Cranston, W. I., Hellon, R. F., Luff, R. H., Rawlins, M. D. & Rosendorff, C. (1970). Observations on the mechanism of salicylate-induced antipyresis. *J. Physiol. (Lond)*, **210**, 593–600.

Cranston, W. I., Duff, G. W., Hellon, R. F. & Mitchell, D. (1976a). Effect of a prostaglandin antagonist on the pyrexias caused by PGE_2 and leucocyte pyrogen in rabbits. *J. Physiol. (Lond)*, **256**, 120–1P.

Cranston, W. I., Duff, G. W., Hellon, R. F., Mitchell, D. & Townsend, Y. (1976b). Evidence that brain prostaglandin synthesis is not essential in fever. *J. Physiol. (Lond)*, **259**, 239–49.

Cranston, W. I., Hellon, R. F. & Townsend, Y. (1980). Suppression of fever in rabbits by a protein synthesis inhibitor, Anisomycin. *J. Physiol. (Lond)*, **305**, 337–44.

Cranston, W. I., Hellon, R. F. & Townsend, Y. (1982). Further observations on the suppression of fever in rabbits by intracerebral action of anisomycin. *J. Physiol. (Lond)*, **322**, 441–5.

Cranston, W. K., Salvador, U. W. & Wheeler, H. O. (1959). The relationship between pyrogen-induced renal vasodilation and circulating pyrogenic substances. *Clin. Sci.*, **18**, 579–85.

Cridland, R. A. & Kasting, N. W. (1992). A critical role for central vasopressin in regulation of fever during bacterial infection. *Amer. J. Physiol.*, **263**, R1235–40.

Currie, J. (1798). *Medical Reports on the Effects of Water Cold and Warm as a Remedy in Fever and other Diseases.* Printed by J. M'Creery for Messrs. Cadell Jun. and Davies, London; and Mr. Creech, Edinburgh. Second Edition. Liverpool. pp. 151–2.

Cushing, H. (1931). The reaction to posterior pituitary extract (Pituitrin) when introduced into the cerebral ventricles. *Proc. Natl. Acad. Sci. (USA)*, **17**, 163–76.

Dascalu, V., Fewell, J. E. & Kondo, C. S. (1989).Carotid-denervation alters the febrile response to bacterial pyrogen in unanaesthetized young lambs. *J. Physiol. (Lond)*, **417**, 18P.

Dascombe, M. J. (1986). Prostanoids in fever: direct evidence for a central source. In *Homeostasis and Thermal Stress*, ed. K. E. Cooper, P. Lomax & E. Schönbaum, pp. 84–7. Karger, Basel.

Dashwood, M. R. & Feldberg, W. (1977). Endotoxin fever, prostaglandin and anesthesia. In *Drugs, Biogenic Amines and Body Temperature*, ed. K. E. Cooper, P. Lomax & E. Schönbaum, pp. 145–52. Karger, Basel.

Davatelis, G., Wolpe, S. D., Sherry, B., Dayer, J. M., Chicheportiche, R. & Cerami, A. (1989). Macrophage inflammatory protein-1: a prostaglandin – independent endogenous pyrogen. *Science*, **243**, 1066–88.

Davidson, J., Milton, A. S. & Rotondo, D. (1992). α-Melanocyte-stimulating hormone suppresses fever and increases in plasma levels of prostaglandin E_2 in the rabbit. *J. Physiol. (Lond)*, **451**, 491–502.

De Luca, B., Monda, M., Pellicano, M. P. & Zenga, A. (1987). Cortical control of thermogenesis induced by lateral hypothalamic lesion and overeating. *Am. J. Physiol.*, **253** (*Regulatory Integrative Comp. Physiol.*, **23**), R626–R633.

De Luca, B., Monda, M., Amaro, S. & Pellicano, M. P. (1989). Thermogenic changes following frontal neocortex stimulation. *Brain Res. Bull.*, **22**, 1003–7.

De Vries, G. J., Buijs, R. M., Van Leeuwen, F. W., Caff, A. R. & Swaab, D. F. (1985). The vasopressinergic innervation of the brain in normal and castrated rats. *J. Comp. Neurol.*, **233**, 236–54.

Delgado, J. M. R. & Livingstone, R. B. (1948). Some respiratory, vascular and thermal responses to stimulation of orbital surface of frontal lobe. *J. Neurophysiol.*, **11**, 39–55.

Derijk, R. & Berkenbosch, F. (1992). Development and application of a radioimmunoassay to detect interleukin-1 in rat peripheral circulation. *Amer. J. Physiol.*, **263**, E1092–8.

Dey, P. K., Feldberg, W., Gupta, K. P. & Wendtlandt, S. (1975). Lipid A fever in cats. *J. Physiol. (Lond).*, **253**, 103–19.

Dinarello, C. A. (1988). Biology of interleukin-1. *FASEB J.*, **2**, 108–15.

Dinarello, C. A., Renfer, L. & Wolff, S. M. (1977). Human leukocytic pyrogen: purification and development of a radioimmunoassay. *Proc. Natl. Acad. Sci. USA*, **74**, 4624–7.

Dinarello, C. A., Weiner, P. & Wolff, S. M. (1978). Radiolabelling and disposition in rabbits of purified human leucocytic pyrogen. *Clin. Res.*, **26**, 522A.

Dinarello, C. A., Bernheim, H. A., Duff, G. W., Le, H. V., Nagabhushan, T. L., Hamilton, N. C. & Coceani, F. (1984). Mechanisms of fever induced by recombinant human interferon. *J. Clin. Invest.*, **74**, 906–13.

Dinarello, C. A., Cannon, J. G., Wolff, S. M., Bernheim, H. A., Beutler, B., Cerami, A., Figari, I. S., Palladino, M. A. & O'Connor, J. V. (1986). Tumor necrosis factor (cachectin) is an endogenous pyrogen and induces production of interleukin-1. *J. Exptl. Med.*, **163**, 1433–50.

Dinarello, C. A., Cannon, J. G., Mancilla, J., Bishai, I., Lees, J. & Coceani, F. (1991). Interleukin-6 as an endogenous pyrogen: induction of prostaglandin E_2 in brain but not in peripheral blood mononuclear cells. *Brain Res.*, **562**, 199–206.

Disturnal, J. E., Veale, W. L. & Pittman, Q. J. (1985). Electrophysiological analysis of potential arginine vasopressin projections to the ventral septal area of the rat. *Brain Res.*, **342**, 162–7.

Disturnal, J. E., Veale, W. L. & Pittman, Q. J. (1986). Thermoresponsive units in the ventral septal area of the rat brain: evidence for involvement in AVP antipyresis. In *Homeostasis and Thermal Stress*, ed. K. E. Cooper, P. Lomax, E. Schönbaum & W. L. Veale, pp. 140–4. Karger, Basel.

Disturnal, J. E., Veale, W. L. & Pittman, Q. J. (1987). Modulation by arginine vasopressin of glutamate excitation in the ventral septal area of the rat brain. *Can. J. Physiol. Pharmacol.*, **65**, 30–5.

Dorsa, D. M., Petracca, F. M., Baskin, D. G. & Cornett, L. E. (1984). Localization and characterization of vasopressin-binding sites in the amygdala of the rat brain. *J. Neurosci.*, **4**, 1764–70.

Downey, J. A., Mottram, R. F. & Pickering, G. W. (1964). The location by regional cooling of central temperature receptors in the conscious rabbit. *J. Physiol. (Lond)*, **170**, 415–41.

Dragunow, M. & Faull, R. (1989). The use of c-fos as a metabolic marker in neuronal pathway tracing. *J. Neurosci. Methods*, **29**, 261–5.

Eisenman, J. S. (1969). Pyrogen induced changes in thermosensitivity of septal and preoptic neurons. *Amer. J. Physiol.*, **216**, 330–4.

Eisenman, J. S. (1972). Unit activity studies of thermosensitive neurons. In *Essays on Temperature Regulation*, ed. J. Bligh, & R. E. Moore, pp. 55–69. North Holland Publishing Company, Amsterdam.

Eisenman, J. S. (1974). Depression of preoptic thermosensitivity by bacterial pyrogen in rabbits. *Amer. J. Physiol.*, **227**, 1067–73.

Eisenman, J. S. (1982). Electrophysiology of the anterior hypothalamus: thermoregulation and fever. In *Pyretics and Antipyretics*, ed. A. S. Milton, pp. 187–217. Springer-Verlag, Berlin.

Eliasson, S. & Ström, G. (1950). On the localization in the cat of hypothalamic and cortical structures influencing cutaneous blood flow. *Acta Physiol. Scand.*, **20** (Suppl. 70), 113–18.

Elin, R. J. & Wolff, S. M. (1974). The role of iron in nonspecific resistance to infection induced by endotoxin. *J. Immunol.*, **112**, 737–45.

Euler, C., von (1961). Physiology and pharmacology of temperature regulation. *Pharmacol. Rev.*, **13**, 361–98.

Farrar, W. L., Kilian, P. L., Ruff, M. R., Hill, J. M. & Pert, B. (1987). Visualization and characterization of interleukin-1 receptors in brain. *J. Immunol.*, **139**, 459–63.

Federico, P., Willcox, B. J., Cooper, K. E. & Veale, W. L. (1992a). Vasopressin induced antipyresis and convulsive like activity in the medial amygdaloid nucleus. In *Thermoregulation: The Pathological Basis of Clinical Disorders*, ed. P. Lomax & E. Schönbaum, pp. 19–24. Karger, Basel.

Federico, P., Malkinson, T. J., Cooper, K. E., Pittman, Q. J. & Veale, W. L. (1992b). Vasopressin perfusion within the medial amygdaloid nucleus attenuates prostaglandin fever in the urethane-anesthetized rat. *Brain Res.*, **587**, 319–26.

Federico, P., Veale, W. L. & Pittman, Q. J. (1992c). Vasopressin-induced antipyresis in the medial amygdaloid nucleus of conscious rats. *Amer. J. Physiol.*, **262**, R901–8.

Feldberg, W. (1975). Body temperature and fever: changes in our views during the last decade. *Proc. Roy. Soc. Lond.*, **191**, 191–229.

Feldberg, W. & Gupta, K. P. (1973). Pyrogen fever and prostaglandin activity in cerebrospinal fluid. *J. Physiol. (London)*, **228**, 41–53.

Feldberg, W. & Myers, R. D. (1963). A new concept of temperature regulation by amines in the hypothalamus. *Nature*, **200**, 1325.

Feldberg, W. & Myers, R. D. (1965). Changes in temperature produced by micro-injections of amines into the anterior hypothalamus of the cat. *J. Physiol. (Lond)*, **177**, 239–45.

Feldberg, W. & Saxena, P. N. (1971a). Fever produced by prostaglandin E_1. *J. Physiol. (Lond)*, **217**, 547–56.

Feldberg, W. & Saxena, P. N. (1971b). Further studies on prostaglandin E_1 fever in cats. *J. Physiol. (Lond)*, **219**, 739–45.

Feldberg, W., Gupta, K. P., Milton, A. S. & Wendtlandt, S. (1973). Effect of pyrogen and antipyretics on prostaglandin activity in cisternal CSF of unanaesthetized cats. *J. Physiol. (Lond)*, **234**, 279–303.

Ferguson, A. V., Veale, W. L. & Cooper, K. E. (1981). Age related differences in the febrile response of the New Zealand White rabbit to endotoxin. *Can. J. Physiol. Pharmacol.*, **59**, 613–14.

Fessler, J. H., Cooper, K. E., Cranston, W. I. & Vollum, R. L. (1961). Observations on the production of pyrogenic substances by rabbit and human leucocytes. *J. Exptl. Med.*, **113**, 1127–40.

Fielden, L. J., Waggoner, J. P., Perrin, M. R. & Hickman, G. C. (1990). Thermoregulation in the Namib Desert Golden Mole, *Erimitalpa granti Namibensis* (Chrysochloridæ). *J. Arid Environ.*, **18**, 221–37.

Fontana, A., Weber, E. & Dayer, J. M. (1984). Synthesis of interleukin-1/endogenous pyrogen in the brain of endotoxin treated mice: a step in fever induction. *J. Immunol.*, **133**, 1696–8.

Fox, R. H. & Hilton, S. M. (1958). Bradykinin formation in human skin as a factor in heat vasodilatation. *J. Physiol. (Lond)*, **142**, 219–32.

Fox, R. H. & MacPherson, R. K. (1954). The regulation of body temperature during fever. *J. Physiol. (Lond)*, **125**, 21P.

François-Franck, C. E. (1876). Du volume des organes en rapport avec la circulation du sang. *Trav. du Lab. de Marey*, **2**, 1.

Freund-Mercier, M. J., Stoeckel, M. E., Dietl, J. M. & Richard, Ph. (1988). Quantitative autoradiographic mapping of neurohypophysial hormone binding sites in the rat forebrain and pituitary gland – 1, Characterization of different types of binding sites and their distribution on the Long-Evans strain. *Neurosci.*, **26**, 261–72.

Fujimoto, N., Kaneko, T., Eguchi, N., Urade, Y., Mizuno, N. & Hayaishi, O. (1992). Biochemical and immunohistological demonstration of a tightly bound form of PGE_2 in the rat brain. *Neuroscience*, **49**, 591–606.

Fulton, J. F. (1949). Cerebral cortex: Autonomic representation in precentral motor cortex. In *Physiology of the Nervous System*, 3rd edn., ed. J. F. Fulton, pp. 468–84. Oxford University Press, New York.

Fyda, D. M., Cooper, K. E. & Veale, W. L. (1989). Indomethacin-induced antipyresis in the rat: role of vasopressin receptors. *Brain Res.*, **494**, 307–14.

Fyda, D. M., Cooper, K. E. & Veale, W. L. (1991). Nucleus tractus solitarii lesions alter the metabolic and hyperthermic response to central prostaglandin E_1 in the rat. *J. Physiol. (Lond)*, **442**, 337–49.

Fyda, D. M., Mathieson, W. B., Cooper, K. E. & Veale, W. L. (1990). The effectiveness of arginine vasopressin and sodium salicylate as antipyretics in the Brattleboro rat. *Brain Res.*, **512**, 243–7.

Gallego, R., Eyzaguirre, C. & Monti-Bloch, L. (1979). Thermal and osmotic responses of arterial receptors. *J. Neurophysiol.*, **42**, 665–80.

Gander, G. W. & Milton, A. S. Quoted in Milton, A. S. (1976). Modern views on the pathogenesis of fever and the mode of action of antipyretic drugs. *J. Pharm. Pharmac.*, **28**, 393–9.

Gerbrandy, J., Cranston, W. I. & Snell, E. S. (1954a). The initial process in the action of bacterial pyrogens in man. *Clin. Sci.*, **13**, 453–9.

Gerbrandy, J., Snell, E. S. & Cranston, W. I. (1954b). Oral, rectal and oesophageal temperatures in relation to central temperature control in man. *Clin. Sci.*, **13**, 615–24.

Gerhardt, C. von. (1853). Untersuchungen über die wasserfreien organischen Sären. *Justus Liebig Annals Chem.*, **87**, 149–78.

Gerland, H. (1852). New formation of salicylic acid. *J. Chem. Soc.*, **5**, 133.

Gery, I. & Waksman, B. H. (1972). Potentiation of the T-lymphocyte response to mitogens II. The cellular source of potentiating mediators. *J. Exptl. Med.*, **136**, 143–55.

Gisolfi, C. V., Wall, P. T. & Mitchell, W. R. (1983). Thermoregulatory responses to central injections of excess calcium in monkeys. *Amer. J. Physiol.*, **245**, R76–R82.

Gisolfi, C. V., Lamb, D. R. & Nadel, E. R. (eds.) (1993). *Perspectives in Exercise Science and Sports Medicine*, Vol.6, *Exercise, Heat, and Thermoregulation*. Brown & Benchmark, Dubuque, USA.

Glyn, J. R. & Lipton, J. M. (1981). Hypothermic and antipyretic effects of centrally administered ACTH 1-24 and α-melanotropin. *Peptides*, **2**, 177–87.

Glyn-Ballinger, J. R., Bernadini, G. L. & Lipton, J. M. (1983). α-MSH injected into the septal region reduces fever in rabbits. *Peptides*, **4**, 199–203.

Goddard, G. V. (1979). The kindling model of limbic epilepsy. In *Limbic Epilepsy and the Discontrol Syndrome*, ed. M. Girgis & L. G. Kiloh, pp. 107–16. North Holland Biomedical Press, Elsevier.

Goelst, K., Mitchell, D., MacPhail, A. P., Cooper, K. E. & Laburn, H. (1992). Fever response of sheep in the peripartum period to Gram-negative and Gram-positive pyrogens. *Pflügers Arch.*, **420**, 259–63.

Goldring, W., Chassis, H., Ranges, H. A. & Smith, H. W. (1941). Effective renal blood flow in subjects with essential hypertension. *J. Clin. Invest.*, **20**, 637.

Goodman, L. S. & Gilman, A. (1975). *The Pharmacological Basis of Therapeutics*. 5th edn. Macmillan Publishing Co. Inc., Toronto.

Gottschlich, K. W., Werner, J. & Schingnitz, G. (1984). Thermoafferent signal processing in rats: an electrophysiological analysis of midbrain influences on thermoresponsive neurons in the ventrobasal thalamus. *Pflügers Arch.*, **401**, 91–6.

Grant, R. & Whalen, W. J. (1953). Latency of pyrogen fever. Appearance of fast acting pyrogen in blood of febrile animals and in plasma incubated with bacterial pyrogen. *Amer. J. Physiol.*, **173**, 47–54.

Grayson, J. (1951). Observations on the temperature of the human rectum. *Br. Med. J.*, **2**, 1379.

Greenfield, A. D. M. (1960a). Electromechanical methods: Venous occlusion plethysmography, In *Methods in Medical Research*, vol. 8, pp. 293–301. Year Book Publishers Inc., Chicago.

Greenfield, A. D. M. (1960b). Peripheral blood flow by calorimetry. In *Methods in Medical Research*, vol. 8, pp. 302–7. Year Book Publishers Inc., Chicago.

Greisman, S. E., Carozzi, F. A. & Dixon Hills, H, Jr. (1963). Mechanisms of endotoxin tolerance. Relationship between tolerance and reticuloendothelial system phagocytic activity in the rabbit. *J. Exptl. Med.*, **117**, 663–74.

Gross, M. & Greenberg, L. A. (1948). *The Salicylates, a Critical Review*. Hillhouse Press, New Haven.

Grundmann, M. J. (1969). Studies on the action of antipyretic substances. D.Phil. Thesis. University of Oxford. England.

Hacker, M. R., Rothenburg, B. A. & Kluger, M. I. (1981). Plasma iron, copper and zinc in lizard Dipsosaurus dorsalis: effects of bacterial infection. *Amer. J. Physiol.*, **240**, R272–5.

Halvorson, T. & Thornhill, J. (1993). Posterior hypothalamic stimulation of anesthetized normothermic and hypothermic rats evokes thermogenesis. *Brain Res.*, **610**, 208–15.

Hammel, H. T., Hardy, J. D. & Fusco, M. M. (1960). Thermoregulatory responses to hypothalamic cooling in unanesthetized dogs. *Amer. J. Physiol.*, **198**, 481–6.

Hanson, D. F., Murphy, P. A. & Windle, B. E. (1980). Failure of rabbit neutrophils to secrete endogenous pyrogen when stimulated with staphylococci. *J. Exptl. Med.*, **151**, 1360–71.

Harvey, C. A. & Milton, A. S. (1974). The effect of parachlorophenylalanine on the response of the conscious cat to intravenous and intraventricular bacterial pyrogen and to intraventricular prostaglandin E_1. *J. Physiol. (Lond)*, **236**, 14–15P.

Hashimoto, M. (1915). Fieberstudien. 1. Mitteilung: Über die spezifische Uberempfindlichkeit des warmentrums an sensibilisierten Tieren. *Arch. exp. Path. Pharmak.*, **78**, 370–93.

Hashimoto, M., Ishikawa, Y., Yokoto, S., Goto, F., Bando, T., Sakakibara, Y. & Iriki, M. (1991). Action site of circulating interleukin-1 on the rabbit brain. *Brain Res.*, **540**, 217–23.

Heap, R. B., Silver, A. & Walters, D. E. (1981). Effects of pregnancy on the febrile response in sheep. *Q. J. Exp. Physiol.*, **66**, 129–44.

Hellon, R. F. (1967). Thermal stimulation of hypothalamic neurones in unanaesthetized rabbits. *J. Physiol. (Lond)*, **193**, 381–95.

Hellon, R. F. (1972). Central thermoreceptors and thermoregulation. In *Handbook of Sensory Physiology*, ed. E. Neil, vol.3, pp. 161–86. Springer, Heidelberg.

Hellon, R. F. & Townsend, Y. (1983). Mechanisms of fever. *Pharmac. Ther.*, **19**, 211–44.

Hellon, R., Townsend, Y., Laburn, H. P. & Mitchell, D. (1991). Mechanisms of fever. In *Thermoregulation Pathology, Pharmacology and Therapy. International Encyclopedia of Pharmacology and Therapeutics*, section 132, ed. E. Schönbaum & P. Lomax, pp. 19–54. Pergamon Press, Oxford.

Hemingway, A. (1963). Shivering. *Physiol. Rev.*, **43**, 397–422.

Hensel, H. (1973a). Neural processes in thermoregulation. *Physiol. Rev.*, **53**, 948–1017.

Hensel, H. (1973b). Cutaneous thermoreceptors. In *Handbook of Sensory Physiology*, vol.II, *Somatosensory System*, ed. A. Iggo, p. 86. Springer Verlag, Berlin.

Hensel, H. (1981). *Thermoreception and Temperature Regulation*. Monographs of the Physiological Society No.38, p. 34. Academic Press, New York.

Herlitz, G. (1941). Studien über die sogenannten initialen Fieberkrämpfe bei Kindern. *Acta Paediatr. Scand.* (Suppl.1), 29.

Himms-Hagen, J. (1990). Brown adipose tissue thermogenesis: role in thermoregulation, energy regulation and obesity. In *Thermoregulation, Physiology and Biochemistry. International Encyclopedia of Pharmacology and Therapeutics*, section 131, ed. E. Schönbaum, & P. Lomax, pp. 327–414. Pergamon Press, Oxford.

Hockaday, T. D. R., Cranston, W. I., Cooper, K. E. & Mottram, R. F. (1962). Temperature regulation in chronic hypothermia. *Lancet*, **2**, 428–32.

Hori, T. & Harada, Y. (1976). Midbrain neuronal responses to local and spinal cord temperatures. *Amer. J. Physiol.*, **231**, 1573–8.

Hori, T., Shibata, M., Nakashima, T., Yamasaki, M., Asami, A., Asami,

T. & Koga, H. (1988). Effects of interleukin-1 and arachidonate on the preoptic and anterhypothalamic neurons. *Brain Res. Bull.*, **20**, 75–82.

Hosoya, Y., Sugiura, Y., Okado, N., Loewy, A. D. & Kohno, K. (1991). Descending input from the hypothalamic paraventricular nucleus to sympathetic preganglionic neurons in the rat. *Exp. Brain Res.*, **85**, 10–20.

Huxley, T. H. (1860). In *Life and Letters of Thomas Henry Huxley*, ed. Leonard Huxley, p. 219. MacMillan & Co. Ltd., London (1900).

Huxley, T. H. (1873). Biogenesis and abiogenesis. Presidential address to the British Association for the Advancement of Science, 1870. In *Critiques and Addresses*, p. 229. MacMillan & Co. Ltd., London.

Iggo, A. (1969). Cutaneous thermoreceptors in primates and non-primates. *J. Physiol. (Lond)*, **200**, 403–30.

Iggo, A. & Paintal, A. S. (1977). The metabolic dependence of primate cutaneous cold receptors. *J. Physiol. (Lond)*, **272**, 40–1P.

Imai-Matsumura, K. & Nakayama, I. (1987). The central efferent mechanism of brown adipose tissue thermogenesis induced by preoptic cooling. *Can. J. Physiol. Pharmacol.*, **65**, 1299–303.

Ingram, D. L. & Legge, K. F. (1972). The influence of deep body temperatures and skin temperatures on respiratory frequency in the pig. *J. Physiol. (Lond)*, **220**, 283–96.

Ingram, D. L., McLean, J. A. & Whittow, G. C. (1963). The effect of heating the hypothalamus and the skin on the rate of moisture vaporization from the skin of the ox (*Bos taurus*). *J. Physiol. (Lond)*, **169**, 394–403.

Jackson, D. (1967). A hypothalamic region responsive to localized injections of pyrogens. *J. Neurophysiol.*, **30**, 536–602.

Janský, L. (1979). Heat production. In *Body Temperature, Regulation, Drug Effects and Therapeutic Implications*, ed. P. Lomax & E. Schönbaum, pp. 89–117. Marcel Dekker Inc., New York.

Johnson, A. & Loewy, A. D. (1990). Circumventricular organs and their role in visceral functions. In *Central Regulations of Autonomic Functions*, ed. A. D. Loewy & K. M. Spyer, Oxford University Press, Oxford.

Johnson, R. H. & Spalding, J. M. K. (1974). *Disorders of the Autonomic Nervous System*, pp. 2–4. Blackwell Scientific Publications, Oxford.

Kaiser, H. K. & Wood, W. B. (1962). Studies on the pathogenesis of fever. IX. The production of endogenous pyrogen by polymorphonuclear leucocytes. *J. Exp. Med.*, **115**, 27–36.

Kampschmidt, R. F. (1978). Leucocytic endogenous mediator. *J. Reticuloendothel. Soc.*, **23**, 287–97.

Kampschmidt, R. F. & Upchurch, H. F. (1970). The effect of endogenous pyrogen on the plasma zinc concentration of the rat. *Proc. Soc. Exp. Biol. Med.*, **134**, 1150–2.

Kandasamy, S. B. & Williams, B. A. (1984). Hypothermic and antipyretic effect of ACTH (1-24) and α-melanotropin in guinea pigs. *Neuropharmacology*, **23**, 49–51.

Karunaweera, N. D., Grau, G. E., Gamage, P., Carter, R. & Mendis, K. N. (1992). Dynamics of fever and serum levels of tumor necrosis factor are closely associated during paroxysms Plasmodium vivax malaria. *Proc. Natl. Acad. Sci. USA.*, **89**, 3200–3.

Kasting, N. W. (1980). An antipyretic system in the brain and the role of vasopressin. PhD. Thesis. The University of Calgary, Calgary, Canada.

Kasting, N. W & Martin, J. B. (1983). Changes in immunoreactive vasopressin concentrations in brain regions of the rat in response to endotoxin. *Brain Res.*, **258**, 127–32.

Kasting, N. W., Veale, W. L. & Cooper, K. E. (1980). Convulsive and hypothermic effects of vasopressin in the brain of the rat. *Can. J. Physiol. Pharmacol.*, **58**, 316–19.

Kasting, N. W., Veale, W. L., Cooper, K. E. & Lederis, K. (1981). Effect of hemorrhage on fever: The putative role of vasopressin. *Can. J. Physiol. Pharmacol.*, **59**, 324–8.

Kawano, H. & Masuko, S. (1992). Met-enkephalin-Arg^6-Gly^7-Leu^8- and substance P-containing projections from the nucleus preopticus medianus to the paraventricular hypothalamic nucleus. *Neuroscience Letters*, **148**, 211–15.

Kawasaki, H., Moriyama, M., Ohtani, Y., Neitoh, M. & Tanaka, A. (1989). Analysis of endotoxin fever in rabbits by using a monoclonal antibody to tumor necrosis factor (Cachectin). *Infection and Immunity*, **57**, 3131–5.

Kerslake, D. McK. (1972). *The Stress of Hot Environments*. Cambridge University Press, Cambridge.

Kerslake, D. McK. & Cooper, K. E. (1950). Vasodilatation in the hand in response to heating the skin elsewhere. *Clin. Sci.*, **9**, 31–47.

King, M. K. & Wood, W. B. (1958). Studies on the pathogenesis of fever. IV. The site of action of leucocytic and circulating endogenous pyrogen. *J. Exp. Med.*, **107**, 291–303.

Kleinebeckel, D. & Klussman, F. W. (1990). Shivering. In *Thermoregulation, Physiology and Biochemistry. International Encyclopedia of Pharmacology and Therapeutics*, section 131, ed. E. Schönbaum & P. Lomax, pp. 235–53. Pergamon Press, Oxford.

Kluger, M. J. (1977). Fever in the frog Hyla cinerea. *J. Therm. Biol.*, **2**, 79–81.

Kluger, M. J. (1979). *Fever its Biology, Evolution and Function*. Princeton University Press, Princeton, New Jersey.

Kluger, M. J. (1981). Is fever a nonspecific host defense response? In *The Physiologic and Metabolic Responses of the Host*, ed. M. C. Powanda & P. G. Canonico, North Holland Biomedical Press, Elsevier.

Kluger, M. J. (1986). Is fever beneficial? *Yale J. Biol. Med.*, **59**, 89–95.

Kluger, M. J. (1991a). Fever: role of pyrogens and cryogens. *Physiol. Rev.*, **71**, 93–127.

Kluger, M. J. (1991b). Fever and Sepsis. In *Obesity and Cachexia*, ed. N. J. Rothwell & M. J. Stock, pp. 159–73. John Wiley & Sons Ltd.

Kluger, M. J. (1992). The role of IL-1, TNF, and IL-6 in fever in the rat. In *Neuroimmunology of Fever*, ed. T. Bartfai & D. Ottoson, pp. 87–96. Pergamon Press, Oxford.

Kluger, M. J. & Vaughn, L. K. (1978). Fever and survival in rabbits infected with Pasteurella multocida. *J. Physiol. (Lond)*, **282**, 243–51.

Kluger, M. J., Ringler, D. H. & Anver, M. R. (1975). Fever and survival. *Science*, **188**, 166–8.

Kluger, M. J., O'Reilly, B., Shope, T. R. & Vander, A. J. (1987). Further evidence that stress hyperthermia is a fever. *Physiol. & Behav.*, **39**, 763–6.

Kolbe, H. & Lautemann, E. (1860). Über die Constitution und Basicität der

Salicylsäure. *Justus Liebigs Annals Chem.*, **115**, 157–206.

Komaki, G., Arimura, A. & Koves, K. (1992). Effect of intravenous injection of IL-1 beta on PGE$_2$ levels in several brain areas as determined by microdialysis. *Amer. J. Physiol.*, **262**, E246–51.

Komáromi, I., Malkinson, T. J., Veale, W. L., Rosenbaum, G., Cooper, K. E. & Pittman, Q. J. (1994). The effect of potassium-induced cortical spreading depression on prostaglandin-induced fever in conscious and urethane anesthetized rats. *Can. J. Physiol. Pharm.*, **72**, 716–21.

Kruse, H., Van Wimersma Greidanus, Tj. B. & De Wied, D. (1977). Barrel rotation induced by vasopressin and related peptides in rats. *Pharmacol. Biochem. Behav.*, **7**, 311–13.

Laburn, H., Mitchell, D. & Rosendorff, C. (1977). Effects of prostaglandin antagonism on sodium arachidonate fever in rabbits. *J. Physiol. (Lond)*, **267**, 559–70.

Laburn, H. P., Mitchell, D., Kenedi, E. & Louw, G. N. (1981). Pyrogens fail to produce fever in a cordylid lizard. *Amer. J. Physiol.*, R198–202.

Landgraf, R., Malkinson, T. J., Veale, W. L., Lederis, K. & Pittman, Q. J. (1990). Vasopressin and oxytocin in rat brain in response to prostaglandin fever. *Amer. J. Physiol.*, R1056–62.

Landy, M. (1971). Discussion. In *Pyrogens and Fever*, ed. G. E. W. Wolstenholme & J. Birch, p. 213. Churchill Livingstone, Edinburgh.

Le Gros Clark, W. E. & Meyer, M. (1950). Anatomical relationship between the cerebral cortex and hypothalamus. *Brit. Med. Bull.*, **6**, 341–4.

Lechan, R. M., Toni, R., Clark, B. D., Cannon, J. G., Shaw, A. R., Dinarello, C. A. & Reichlin, S. (1990). Immunoreactive interleukin-1β localization in the rat forebrain. *Brain Res.*, **514**, 135–40.

Lederis, K., Pittman, Q. J., Kasting, N. W., Veale, W. L. & Cooper, K. E. (1982). Central neuromodulatory role for vasopressin in antipyresis and in febrile convulsions. *Biomed. Res.*, **3**, 1–5.

Lefèvre, J. (1911). *Chaleur animale et Bioénergétique*, p. 354. Masson, Paris.

LeMay, L. G., Otterness, I. G., Vander, A. J. & Kluger, M. J. (1990). In vivo evidence that the rise in plasma IL 6 following injection of a fever-inducing dose of LPS is mediated by IL-1β. *Cytokine*, **2**, 199–204.

Lennox-Buchtal, M. A. (1976). A summing up: clinical session. In *Brain Dysfunction in Infantile Febrile Convulsions*, ed. M. A. B. Brazier & F. Coceani, pp. 327–51. Raven Press, New York.

Lepe-Ziniga, J. L. & Gery, I. (1984). Production of intra- and extracellular interleukin-1 (IL-1) by human monocytes. *Clin. Immunol. Immunopath.*, **31**, 220–30.

Lewis, T. (1930). Observations upon the reactions of the vessels of the human skin to cold. *Heart*, **15**, 177–208.

Liebermeister, C. (1871). Ueber Wärmeregulirung und Fieber. *Sammlung klinischer Vorträge in Verbindung mit deutschen Klinikern, herausgegeben von Richard Volkman*, No. 19. Druck und Verlag von Breitkopf und Härtel, Leipzig.

Lipton, J. M. & Glyn, J. R. (1980). Central administration of peptides alters thermoregulation in the rabbit. *Peptides*, **1**, 15–18.

Lipton, J. M. & Murphy, M. T. (1983). Aging enhances the antipyretic effect of α-MSH and the hyperthermic effect of central β-endorphin. In *Environment, Drugs and Thermoregulation*, ed. P. Lomax & E. Schönbaum, Karger, Basel.

Lipton, J. M. & Trzcinka, G. P. (1976). Persistence of febrile response after

AH/POA lesions in squirrel monkeys. *Amer. J. Physiol.*, **231**, 1638–48.

Lipton, J. M., Kirkpatrick, J. & Rosenberg, R. N. (1977). Hypothermia and persisting capacity to develop fever. *Arch. Neurol.*, **34**, 498–504.

Lipton, J. M., Whisenant, J. D., Gean, J. T. & Ticknor, C. B. (1979). Effects on fever of central administration of transport inhibitors. *Brain Res. Bull.*, **4**, 297–300.

Lomedico, P. T., Gubler, U., Hellman, C. P., Dukovich, M., Giri, J. G., Pan, Y. E., Collier, K., Semionow, R., Chua, A. O. & Mizel, S. B. (1984). Cloning and expression of murine interleukin-1 in Escherichia coli. *Nature*, **312**, 458–62.

Long, N. C., Kluger, M. J. & Vander, A. J. (1989). Antiserum against mouse IL-1 does not block stress hypothermia or LPS fever in the rat. In *Thermoregulation: Research and Clinical Applications*, ed. P. Lomax & E. Schönbaum, pp. 78–84. Karger, Basel.

Long, N. C., Vander, A. J., Kunkel, S. L. & Kluger, M. J. (1990a). Antiserum against tumor necrosis factor increases stress hyperthermia in rats. *Amer. J. Physiol.*, **258**, R591–5.

Long, N. C., Kunkel, S. L., Vander, A. J. & Kluger, M. J. (1990b). Antiserum against TNF enhances LPS fever in the rat. *Amer. J. Physiol.*, **258**, R332–7.

Lorin, M. I. (1982). The febrile child. *Clinical Management of Fever and Other Types of Pyrexia*, Chapter 12. John Wiley & Sons, New York.

Luderitz, O., Galanos, C., Lehmann, V., Nurminen, K., Reitschel, E. T., Rosenfelder, G., Simon, M. & Westphal, O. (1973). Lipid A: chemical structure and biological activity. *I. Infect. Dis.*, **128** (Suppl.), 17–29.

Luiten, P. G. M., Horst, G. J. ter, Karst, H. & Steffens, A. B. (1985). The course of paraventricular hypothalamic efferents to autonomic structures in medulla and spinal cord. *Brain Res.*, **329**, 374–8.

Lyons, A. S. & Petrucelli, R. J. (1987). *Medicine an Illustrated History*, p. 454. Abradale Press, Harry N. Abrams, Inc., New York.

Macpherson, R. K. (1959). The effect of fever on temperature regulation in man. *Clin. Sci.*, **18**, 281–7.

Magoun, H. W., Harrison, F., Brobeck, J. R. & Ranson, S. W. (1938). Activation of heat loss mechanism by local heating of the brain. *J. Neurophysiol.*, **1**, 101–14.

Malkinson, T. J., Taylor, P. J. & Cooper, K. E. (1978). Temperature gradients within the human pelvis and the measurement of blood flow during laparoscopy. In *Endoscopy in Gynecology*, pp. 71–5. The proceedings of the third International Congress on Gynecologic Endoscopy, San Francisco, USA. The American Association of Gynecologic Laparoscopists.

Malkinson, T. J., Veale, W. L. & Cooper, K. E. (1985). Fever and intracranial pressure. *Brain Res. Bull.*, **15**, 315–19.

Malkinson, T. J., Bridges, T. E., Lederis, K. & Veale, W. L. (1987). Perfusion of the septum of the rabbit with vasopressin antiserum enhances endotoxin fever. *Peptides*, **8**, 385–9.

Malkinson, T. J., Cooper, K. E. & Veale, W. L. (1988). Physiological changes during thermoregulaton and fever in urethane-anesthetized rats. *Amer. J. Physiol.*, **255**, R73–R81.

Malkinson, T. J., Veale, W. L. & Cooper, K. E. (1993). Intracranial pressures and fever in the rat, rabbit and cat. In *Intracranial Pressure*

VIII, ed. C. J. J. Avezaat, J. H. M. van Eijndhoven, A. I. R. Mass & TH. J. Tans, pp. 198–202. Springer-Verlag, Berlin.

Martin, S., Malkinson, T. J., Veale, W. L. & Pittman, Q. J. (1988). Prostaglandin fever in rats is altered by kainic acid lesions of the ventral septal area. *Brain Res.*, **455**, 196–200.

Martin, S. M., Malkinson, T. J., Veale, W. L. & Pittman, Q. J. (1990). Depletion of brain α-MSH alters prostaglandin and interleukin fevers in rats. *Brain Res.*, **526**, 351–4.

Marx, J., Hilbig, R. & Rahmann, H. (1984). Endotoxin and prostaglandin E_1 fail to induce fever in a teleost fish. *Comp. Biochem. and Physiol.*, **77A**, 483–7.

Mathieson, W. B., Federico, P., Veale, W. L. & Pittman, Q. J. (1989). Single unit activity in the bed nucleus of the stria terminalis during fever. *Brain Res.*, **486**, 49–53.

Matsumura, K., Watanabe, Y., Onoe, H., Watanabe, Y. & Hayaishi, O. (1990). High density of prostaglandin E2 binding sites in the anterior wall of the third ventricle: possible site of its hyperthermic action. *Brain Res.*, **533**, 147–51.

Matsumura, K., Watanabe, Y., Imai-Matsumura, K., Connolly, M., Koyama, Y., Onoe, H. & Watanabe, Y. (1992). Mapping of prostaglandin E_2 binding sites in rat brain using quantitative autoradiography. *Brain Res.*, **581**, 292–8.

Meldrum, B. S. (1976). Secondary pathology of febrile and experimental convulsions. In *Brain Disfunction in Infantile Febrile Convulsions*, ed. M. A. B. Brazier & F. Coceani, pp. 213–22. Raven Press, New York.

Mendelssohn, M. (1902). Récherches sur la thermotaxie des organismes unicellulaire. *J. de Physiol. et de Path. Gen.*, **4**, 393–410.

Mercer, J. B., Jessen, C. & Pierau, Fr.-K. (1978). Thermal stimulation of neurons in the rostral brain stem of conscious goats. *J. Therm. Biol.*, **3**, 5–10.

Merker, G., Blähser, S. & Zeisberger, E. (1980). Reactivity pattern of vasopressin-containing neurons and its relation to the antipyretic reaction in the pregnant guinea pig. *Cell Tissue Res.*, **212**, 47–61.

Michie, H. R., Manogue, K. R., Spriggs, D. R., Revhaug, A., O'Dwyer, S., Dinarello, C. A., Cerami, A., Wolff, S. M. & Wilmore, D. W. (1988). Detection of tumor necrosis factor after endotoxin administration. *New Eng. J. Med.*, **318**, 1481–6.

Miller, F. J. W., Court, S. D. M., Walton, W. S. & Knox, E. J. (1960). Growing up in Newcastle upon Tyne: A continuing study of health and illness in young children within their families. Oxford University Press, Oxford.

Milton, A. S. & Wendlandt, S. (1970). A possible role for prostaglandin E_1 as a modulator for temperature regulation in the central nervous system of the cat. *J. Physiol. (Lond)*, **207**, 76–7P.

Milton, A. S. & Wendlandt, S. (1971). Effects on body temperature of pros-taglandins of the A, E and F series on injection into the third ventricle of unanaesthetized cats and rabbits. *J. Physiol. (Lond)*, **218**, 325–36.

Milton, N. G. N., Hillhouse, E. W. & Milton, A. S. (1992). Activation of the hypothalamo-pituitary-adrenocortical axis in the conscious rabbit by the pyrogen polyinosinic: polycytidylic acid is dependent on corticotrophin-releasing factor-41. *J. Endocrinol.*, **135**, 69–75.

Milton, N. G. N., Hillhouse, E. W. & Milton, A. S. (1993a). Modulation of the prostaglandin responses of conscious rabbits to the pyrogen Polyinosinic: Polycytidylic acid by corticotrophin- releasing factor-41. *J. Endocrinol.*, **138**, 7–11.

Milton, N. G. N., Hillhouse, E. W. & Milton, A. S. (1993b). Does endogenous peripheral arginine vasopressin have a role in the febrile responses of conscious rabbits. *J. Physiol. (Lond)*, **469**, 525–34.

Mitchell, D., Laburn, H., Cooper, K. E., Hellon, R. F., Cranston, W. I. & Townsend, Y. (1986). Is prostaglandin E the neural mediator of the febrile response? The case against a proven obligatory role. *The Yale J. of Biol. Med.*, **59**, 159–68.

Mitchell, D., Laburn, H. P., Matter, M. & McClain, E. (1990). Fever in Namib and other ectotherms. In *Namib Ecology: 25 Years of Namib Research*, ed. M. K. Seely, pp. 179–92. Transvaal Museum Monograph No. 7. Transvaal Museum, Pretoria.

Molenaar, G. J., Berkenbosch, F., van Dam, A. M. & Lugard, C. J. M. E. (1993). Distribution of interleukin-1β immunoreactivity within the porcine hypothalamus. *Brain Res.*, **608**, 169–74.

Moltz, H. (1993). Fever: Causes and consequences. *Neurosci. and Behavior. Revs.*, **17**, 237–69.

Monda, M. & Pittman, Q. J. (1993). Cortical spreading depression blocks prostaglandin E_1 and endotoxin fever in rat. *Amer. J. Physiol.*, R456–9.

Monda, M., Amaro, S., Papa, A. & De Luca, B. (1992). The nervous activation of the interscapular brown adipose tissue during PGE_1 fever is blocked by cortical spreading depression in the rat. *Neurosci. Letters*, Suppl. 43, 575.

Morimoto, A., Murakami, N., Takada, M., Teshirogi, S. & Watanabe, T. (1987). Fever and the acute phase response induced in rabbits by human recombinant Interferon-γ. *J. Physiol. (Lond)*, **391**, 209–18.

Morimoto, A., Murakami, N., Nakamori, T. & Watanabe, T. (1988). Multiple control of fever production in the central nervous system. *J. Physiol. (Lond)*, **397**, 269–80.

Morimoto, A., Murakami, N., Nakamori, T. & Watanabe, T. (1990). Evidence for separate mechanisms of induction of biphasic fever inside and outside the blood-brain barrier in rabbits. *J. Physiol. (Lond)*, **397**, 269–80.

Mott, J. (1963). The effects of baroreceptor and chemoreceptor stimulation on shivering. *J. Physiol. (Lond)*, **166**, 563–86.

Mount, L. E. (1979). *Adaptation to Thermal Environment, Man and His Productive Animals*, pp. 185–90. Edward Arnold, London.

Mrosovsky, N., Molony, L. A., Conn, C. A. & Kluger, M. J. (1989). Anorexic effects of interleukin 1 in the rat. *Amer. J. Physiol.*, **257**, R1315–21.

Murakami, N. (1992). Function of the OVLT as an entrance into the brain for endogenous pyrogens. In *Neuro-Immunology of Fever*, ed. T. Bartfai & D. Ottoson, pp. 107–21. Pergamon Press, Oxford.

Murphy, M. T. & Lipton, J. M. (1982). Peripheral administration of α-MSH reduces fever in older and younger rabbits. *Peptides*, **3**, 775–9.

Murphy, P. A., Chesney, P. J. & Wood, W. B. (1971). Purification of an endogenous pyrogen, with an appendix on assay methods. In *Pyrogens and Fever*, ed. G. E. W. Wolstenholme & J. Birch, pp. 59–79. Churchill Livingstone, Edinburgh.

Myers, R. D. (1969). Temperature regulation: neurochemical systems in the hypothalamus. In *The Hypothalamus*, ed. W. Haymaker, E. Anderson & W. J. H. Nauta. Charles C. Thomas, Springfield.

Myers, R. D. (1982). The role of ions in thermoregulation and fever. In *Pyretics and Antipyretics*, ed. A. S. Milton, pp. 151–86. Springer-Verlag, Berlin.

Myers, R. D. & Tytell, M. (1972). Fever: reciprocal shift in brain sodium to calcium ratio as the set point rises. *Science*, **178**, 765–7.

Myers, R. D. & Veale, W. L. (1971). The role of sodium and calcium ions in the hypothalamus in the control of body temperature of the unanaesthetized cat. *J. Physiol. (Lond)*, **212**, 411–30.

Myers, R. D., Rudy, T. A. & Yaksh, T. L. (1973). Evocation of a biphasic febrile response in the rhesus monkey by intracerebral injection of bacterial endotoxins. *Neuropharmacol.*, **12**, 1195–8.

Myers, R. D., Rudy, T. A. & Yaksh, T. L. (1974). Fever produced by endotoxin injected into the hypothalamus of the monkey and its antagonism by salicylate. *J. Physiol. (Lond)*, **243**, 167–93.

Myhre, K. & Hammel, H. T. (1969). Behavioral regulation of internal temperature in the lizard Tiliqua scincoides. *Amer. J. Physiol.*, **217**, 1490–5.

Myhre, K., Cabanac, M. & Myhre, G. (1977). Fever and behavioural temperature regulation in the frog Rana esculenta. *Acta Physiol. Scand.*, **101**, 219–29.

Nadel, E. R., Horvath, S. M., Dawson, C. A. & Tucker, A. (1970). Sensitivity to central and peripheral thermal stimulation in man. *J. Appl. Physiol.*, **29**, 603–9.

Nakamori, T., Morimoto, A., Yamaguchi, K., Watanabe, T., Long, N. C. & Murakami, N. (1993). Organum vasculosum laminae terminalis (OVLT) is a brain site to produce interleukin-1 beta during fever. *Brain Res.*, **618**, 155–9.

Nakashima, T., Kiyohara, T. & Hori, T. (1991). Tumor necrosis factor-beta specifically inhibits the activity of preoptic warm sensitive neurons in tissue slices. *Neurosci. Lett.*, **128**, 97–100.

Nakayama, T., Eisenman, J. S. & Hardy, J. D. (1961). Single unit activity of anterior hypothalamus during local heating. *Science*, **134**, 560–1.

Nakayama, T., Hammel, H. T., Hardy, J. D. & Eisenman, J. S. (1963). Thermal stimulation of electrical activity of single units of the pre-optic region. *Amer. J. Physiol.*, **204**, 1122–6.

Navarra, P., Pozzoli, G., Brunetti, I., Ragazzoni, E., Besser, M. & Grossman, A. (1992). Interleukin-1 beta and interleukin-6 specifically increase the release of prostaglandin E_2 from rat hypothalamic explants in vitro. *Neuroendocrinology*, **56**, 61–8.

Naylor, A. M. (1987). Central vasopressin and endogenous antipyresis. Ph.D. Thesis. University of Calgary, Canada.

Naylor, A. M., Ruwe, W. D., Kohut, A. F. & Veale, W. L. (1985). Perfusion of vasopressin within the ventral septum of the rabbit suppresses endotoxin fever. *Brain Res. Bull.*, **15**, 209–13.

Naylor, A. M., Pittman, Q. J. & Veale, W. L. (1988). Stimulation of vasopressin release in the ventral septum of the rat suppresses prostaglandin E_1 fever. *J. Physiol. (Lond)*, **399**, 177–89.

Newman, P. P. & Wolstencroft, J. H. (1960). Influence of orbital cortex on blood pressure responses in cat. *J. Neurophysiol.*, **23**, 211–17.

Neyman, C. A. (1936). The effect of artificial fever on the clinical manifestations of syphilis and the treponema pallidum. *Amer. J. Psychiat.*, **93**, 517–27.

Nieto-Sampedro, M. & Berman, M. A. (1987). Interleukin-1 like activity in rat brain: sources, targets, and effect of injury. *J. Neurosci. Res.*, **17**, 214–19.

Nieuwenhuys, R. (1985). *Chemoarchitecture of the Brain*. Springer Verlag, Berlin.

Nissen, R., Bourque, C. W. & Renaud, L. P. (1993). Membrane properties of organum vasculosum lamina terminalis neurons recorded in vitro. *Amer. J. Physiol.*, **264**, R811–15.

Oladehin, A., Barriga-Briceno, J. A. & Blatteis, C. M. (1994). Lipopolysaccharide (LPS)-induced fos expression in the brains of febrile rats. In *Temperature Regulation. Recent Physiological and Pharmacological Advances*, ed. A. S. Milton, pp. 81–5. Birkhäuser Verlag, Basel.

Ono, T., Nishino, H., Sasaka, K., Muramoto, K., Yano, I. & Simpson, A. (1978). *Neuroscience Letters*, **10**, 143–5.

Opp, M., Obál, F. Jr. & Krueger, J. M. (1989). Corticotropin-releasing factor attenuates interleukin-1 induced sleep and fever in rabbits. *Amer. J. Physiol.*, **257**, R528–35.

Ott, I. (1887). The heat-centre in the brain. *J. Nerv. Mental. Dis.*, **14**, 152–62.

Ott, I. (1891). *The Modern Antipyretics: Their Action in Health and Disease*. E. D. Vogel., Easton, Pa.

Ott, I. (1914). *Fever: Its Thermotaxis and Metabolism*. Paul B. Hoeber, New York.

Palkovits, M. & Záborszky, L. (1979). Neural connections of the hypothalamus. In *Handbook of the Hypothalamus*, vol.1, *Anatomy of the Hypothalamus*, ed. P. J. Morgane & J. Panksepp, pp. 379–509. Marcel Dekker, Inc., N. York.

Piani, D., Constam, D. B., Frei, K. & Fontana, A. (1994). Macrophages in the brain: Friends or enemies. *News in Physiological Sciences*, **9**, 80–4.

Pickering, G. W. (1932). The vasomotor regulation of heat loss from the skin in relation to external temperature. *Heart*, **16**, 115–35.

Pickering, G. W. (1961). Fever and pyrogens. *Scientific Basis of Medicine Reviews*, pp. 97–107. University of London, the Athlone Press.

Pillay, V., Savage, N. & Laburn, H. (1993). Interleukin-1 receptor antagonist in newborn babies and pregnant women. *Pflügers Arch.*, **424**, 549–51.

Pinkston, J. O., Bard, P. & Rioch, D. McK. (1934). The responses to changes in environmental temperature after removal of portions of the forebrain. *Amer. J. Physiol.*, **109**, 515–31.

Piria, R. (1838). Sur des nouveaux produits extraits de la salicin. *C. R. Acad. Sci. Paris.*, **6**, 620–4.

Pittman, Q. J. (1976). Fever in foetal and newborn lambs. PhD. Thesis. The University of Calgary, Calgary, Alberta, Canada, T2N 1N4.

Pittman, Q. J., Blume, H. W. & Renaud, L. P. (1981). Connections of the hypothalamic paraventricular nucleus with the neurohypophysis, median eminence, amygdala, lateral septum and midbrain periaqueductal gray: an electrophysiological study in the rat. *Brain Res.*, **215**, 15–28.

Pittman, Q. J., Malkinson, T. J., Kasting, N. W. & Veale, W. L. (1988).

Enhanced fever following castration: possible involvement of brain arginine vasopressin. *Amer. J. Physiol.*, **254**, R513–17.

Poulin, P. & Pittman, Q. J. (1993a). Arginine vasopressin-induced sensitization in brain: facilitated inositol phosphate production without changes in receptor number. *J. Neuroendocrinol.*, **5**, 23–31.

Poulin, P. & Pittman, Q. J. (1993b). Oxytocin pretreatment enhances arginine vasopressin-induced motor disturbances and arginine vasopressin-induced phosphoinositol hydrolysis in rat septum: a cross sensitization phenomenon. *J. Neuroendocrinol.*, **5**, 33–9.

Poulin, P., Lederis, K. & Pittman, Q. J. (1988). Subcellular localization and characterization of vasopressin binding sites in the ventral septal area, lateral septum, and hippocampus of the rat brain. *J. Neurochem.*, **50**, 889–98.

Quan, N., Xin, L. & Blatteis, C. M. (1991). Microdialysis of norepinephrine into preoptic area of guinea pigs: characteristics of hypothermic effect. *Amer. J. Physiol.*, **261**, R378–85.

Ranson, S. W. (1939). *The Anatomy of the Nervous System*. W. B. Saunders, Philadelphia.

Ranson, S. W., Clark, G. & Magoun, H. W. (1939). The effect of hypothalamic lesions on fever induced by intravenous injection of typhoid-paratyphoid vaccine. *J. Lab. Clin. Med.*, **25**, 160–8.

Ravid, R., Swaab, D. F., Van der Woude, T. P. and Boer, G. J. (1986). Immunocytochemically-stained vasopressin binding sites in rat brain. *J. Neurol. Sci.*, **76**, 317–33.

Rawson, R. O. & Quick, K. P. (1976). Intra-abdominal thermoreceptors and the regulation of body temperature in sheep. *Israel J. Med. Sci.*, **12**, 1040–3.

Reaves, T. A. Jr. (1977). Gain of thermosensitive neurons in the preoptic area of the rabbit, Oryctolagus cuniculus. *J. Thermal. Bio.*, **2**, 31–3.

Reaves, T. A. & Heath, J. E. (1975). Interval coding of temperature by CNS neurones in thermoregulation. *Nature*, **257**, 688–90.

Renbourn, E. T. (1960). Body temperature and pulse rate in boys and young men prior to sporting contests. A study in emotional hyperthermia: with a review of the literature. *J. Psychosom. Res.*, **4**, 148–75.

Repin, I. S. & Kratskin, I. I. (1967). An analysis of the hyperthermic mechanism of fever. *Fiziol. Zh. SSSR*, **53**, 1206–11.

Reynolds, W. W., Casterlin, M. E. & Covert, J. B. (1976). Behavioral fever in teleost fishes. *Nature*, **259**, 41–2.

Rezvani, A. H., Denbow, D. M. & Myers, R. D. (1986). a-melanocyte-stimulating hormone infused ICV fails to affect body temperature or endotoxin fever in the cat. *Brain Res. Bull.*, **16**, 99–105.

Richardson, R. P., Rhyne, C. D., Fong, Y., Hesse, D. G., Tracey, K. J., Marano, M.A., Lowry, S. F., Antonacci, A. C. & Calvano, S. E. (1989). Peripheral blood leukocyte kinetics following in vivo lipopolysaccharide (LPS) administration in normal human subjects. *Ann. Surg.*, **210**, 239–45.

Riedel, W. (1990). Mechanics of fever. *J. Basic & Clin. Physiol. & Pharmacol.*, **1**, 291–322.

Riedel, W., Siaplauras, G. & Simon, E. (1973). Intra-abdominal thermosensitivity in the rabbit as compared with spinal thermosensitivity. *Pflügers Arch.* **340**, 50–70.

Rivest, S., Torres, G. & Rivier, C. (1992). Differential effects of central and peripheral injection of interleukin-1β on brain c-fos expression and neuroendocrine functions. *Brain Res.*, **587**, 13–23.

Rosendorff, C. & Mooney, J. J. (1971). Central nervous system sites of action of a purified leucocyte pyrogen. *Amer. J. Physiol.*, **220**, 597–603.

Roth, J., McClellan, J. L., Kluger, M. J. & Zeisberger, E. (1994). Attenuation of fever and release of cytokines after repeated injections of lipopolysaccharide in guinea pigs. *J. Physiol. (Lond)*, **477**, 177–85.

Rothwell, N. J. (1988). Central effects of TNF alpha on thermogenesis and fever in the rat. *Biosci. Rep.*, **8**, 345–52.

Rothwell, N. J. (1989). CRF is involved in the pyrogenic and thermogenic effects of Interleukin-1β in the rat. *Amer. J. Physiol.*, **256**, E111–15.

Rothwell, N. J. (1990). Central activation of thermogenesis by prostaglandins: dependence on CRF. *Horm. Res.*, **22**, 616–18.

Rothwell, N. J. (1992). Ecosinoids, thermogenesis and thermoregulation. *Prostaglandins-Leukot- Essent.-Fatty Acids*, **46**, 1–7.

Rothwell, N. J. (1993). Mechanisms of action of cytokines on fever and thermogenesis. *XXXII Congress of the International Union of Physiological Sciences*, Glasgow, Scotland. Abstract. 316.5/O.

Rotondo, D., Abul, H. T., Milton, A. S. & Davidson, J. (1988). Pyrogenic immunomodulators increase the level of prostaglandin E_2 in the blood simultaneously with the onset of fever. *Eur. J. Pharmacol.*, **154**, 145–52.

Rowley, D., Howard, J. G. & Jenkin, C. R. (1956). The fate of ^{32}P labelled bacterial lipopolysaccharide in laboratory animals. *Lancet*, **1**, 366–7.

Ruwe, W. D., Naylor, A. M. & Veale, W. L. (1985). Perfusion of vasopressin within the rat brain suppresses prostaglandin-E hyperthermia. *Brain Res.*, **338**, 219–24.

Sakata, Y., Morimoto, A. & Murakami, N. (1993). Effects of electrical stimulation or local anesthesia of the rabbit's hypothalamus on the acute phase response. *Brain Res. Bull.*, **31**, 287–92.

Saklatvala, J., Sarsfield, S. T. & Townsend, Y. (1985). Pig interleukin 1: Purification of two immunologically different leukocyte proteins that cause cartilage resorption, lymphocyte activation and fever. *J. Exptl. Med.*, **162**, 1208–22.

Samson, W. K., Lipton, J. M., Zimmer, J. A. & Glyn, J. R. (1981). The effect of fever on central α-MSH concentrations in the rabbit. *Peptides*, **2**, 419–23.

Sanctorii Sanctorii (1701). *Statica Medicina Aphorismorum, Sectiones Septum: cum Commentario Martini Lister*. Sam Smith & Ben, Walford, London.

Saper, C. B. & Breder, C. D. (1992). Endogenous pyrogens in the CNS: role in the febrile response. *Prog. Brain Res.*, **93**, 419–28.

Saper, C. B., Loewy, A. D., Swanson, L. W. & Cowan, W. M. (1976a). Direct hypothalamo-anatomic connections. *Brain Res.*, **117**, 305–12.

Saper, C. B., Swanson, L. W. & Cowan, W. M. (1976b). The efferent connections of the ventromedial nucleus of the hypothalamus of the rat. *J. Comp. Neural.*, **169**, 409–42.

Satinoff, E. (1964). Behavioral thermoregulation in response to local cooling of the rat brain. *Amer. J. Physiol.*, **206**, 1389–94.

Satinoff, E. (1974). Neural integration of thermoregulatory responses. In *Limbic and Autonomic Nervous System Research*, ed. L. V. DiCara, pp. 41–83. Plenum Press, New York.

Schlievert, P. M. & Watson, D. W. (1978). Group A streptococcal pyrogenic endotoxin: Pyrogenicity, alteration of blood-brain barrier, and separation of sites for pyrogenicity and enhancement of lethal endotoxin shock. *Infect. Immunol.*, **21**, 753–63.

Schmidt-Nielsen, K. (1975). *Animal Physiology*. Cambridge University Press, Cambridge.

Schoener, E. P. (1980). Activity of thermoresponsive neurons in fever. In *Fever*, ed. J. M. Lipton, pp. 91–8. Raven Press, New York.

Schoener, E. P. & Wang, S. C. (1976). Effects of locally administered prostaglandin E_1 on anterior hypothalamic neurons. *Brain Res.*, **117**, 157–62.

Schönbaum, E. & Lomax, P. (eds) (1990). *Thermoregulation, Physiology and Biochemistry. International Encyclopedia of Pharmacology and Therapeutics.*. Section 131. Pergamon Press, Oxford.

Scott, I. M., Fertel, R. H. & Boulant, J. A. (1987). Leukocytic pyrogen effects on prostaglandins in hypothalamic tissue slices. *Amer. J. Physiol.*, **253**, R71–6.

Sheagren, T. N., Wolff, S. M. & Shulman, N. R. (1967). Febrile and hematological responses of rhesus monkeys to bacterial endotoxin. *Amer. J. Physiol.*, **212**, 884–90.

Sherrington, C. S. (1924). Notes on temperature after spinal transection with some observations on shivering. *J. Physiol. (Lond)*, **58**, 405–23.

Sheth, U. K. & Borison, H. L. (1960). Central pyrogenic action of Salmonella typhosa lipopolysaccharide injected into the lateral cerebral ventricle in cats. *J. Pharmac. Ther.*, **130**, 411–17.

Shibata, M. & Blatteis, C. M. (1991a). Human recombinant tumor necrosis factor and interferon affect the activity of neurons in the organum vasculosum laminae terminalis. *Brain Res.*, **562**, 323–6.

Shibata, M. & Blatteis, C. M. (1991b). Differential effects of cytokines on thermosensitive neurons in guinea pig preoptic area slices. *Amer. J. Physiol.*, **261**, R1096–103.

Shibata, M., Hori, T., Kiyohara, T., Nakashima, T. & Osaka, T. (1983). Impairment of thermoregulatory cooling behavior by single cortical spreading depression in the rat. *Physiol. and Behav.*, **30**, 599–605.

Shibata, M., Hori, T., Kiyohara, T. & Nakashima, T. (1984). Activity of hypothalamic thermosensitive neurons during cortical spreading depression in the rat. *Brain Res.*, **308**, 255–62.

Shibata, M., Hori, T. & Nagasaka, T. (1985). Effects of single cortical spreading depression on metabolic heat production in the rat. *Physiol. and Behav.*, **34**, 563–7.

Shih, S. T. & Lipton, J. M. (1985). Intravenous α-MSH reduces fever in squirrel monkeys. *Peptides*, **6**, 685–7.

Shih, S. T., Khorram, O., Lipton, J. M. & McCann, S. M. (1986). Central administration of α-MSH antiserum augments fever in the rabbit. *Amer. J. Physiol.*, **250**, R803–6.

Shimada, S. G., Stitt, J. T. & Bernheim, H. A. (1984). Enhancement of the febrile response to endogenous pyrogen in rats by intravenously injected substances that stimulate phagocytosis in reticulo-endothelial system cells. In *Thermal Physiology*, ed. J. R. S. Hales, pp. 551–3. Raven Press, New York.

Shintani, F., Kanba, S., Nakaki, T., Nibuya, M., Kinoshita, N., Suzuki, E., Yagi, G., Kato, R. & Asai, M. (1993). Interleukin-1 beta augments

release of norepinephrine, dopamine, and serotonin in the rat anterior
hypothalamus. *J. Neurosci.*, **13**, 3574–81.

Siegert, R., Philipp-Dormstom, W. K., Radsak, K. & Menzel, H. (1976).
Mechanism of fever induction in rabbits. *Infect. Immunol.*, **14**, 1130–7.

Simon, E. (1974). Temperature regulation: the spinal cord as a site of
extrahypothalamic thermoregulatory functions. *Rev. Physiol. Biochem.
Pharmacol.*, **71**, 1–76.

Simpson, C. W., Ruwe, W. D. & Myers, R. D. (1977). Characterization of
prostaglandin sensitive sites in the monkey hypothalamus mediating
hyperthermia. In *Drugs, Biogenic Amines and Body Temperature*, ed. K.
E. Cooper, P. Lomax & E. Schönbaum, pp. 142–4. Karger, Basel.

Siren, A. L. (1982). Central cardiovascular and thermal effects of
prostaglandin E_2 in rats. *Acta Physiol. Scand.*, **116**, 229–34.

Sirko, S. (1988). Prostanoid release from the hypothalamus in vivo:
implications for the pathogenesis of fever. PhD Thesis, University of
Toronto, Canada.

Sirko, S., Bishai, I. & Coceani, F. (1989). Prostaglandin formation in the
hypothalamus in vivo: effect of pyrogens. *Amer. J. Physiol.*, **256**,
R616–24.

Snell, E. S. (1971). In *Pyrogens and Fever*, ed. G. E. W. Wolstenholme & J.
Birch. Discussion, p. 212. Churchill Livingstone, Edinburgh.

Snell, E. S. & Atkins, E. (1965). The presence of endogenous pyrogen in
normal rabbit tissues. *J. Exptl. Med.*, **121**, 1019–38.

Sofroniew, M. V. & Weindl, A. (1978). Projections from the parvocellular
vasopressin- and neurophysin-containing neurons of the suprachiasmatic
nucleus. *Amer. J. Anat.*, **153**, 391–430.

Stark, R. I., Daniel, S. S., Husain, K. M., James, L. S. & Van de Wiele, R.
L. (1979). Arginine vasopressin during gestation and parturition in sheep
fetus. *Biol. Neonate*, **35**, 235–41.

Stitt, J. T. (1973). Prostaglandin E_1 fever induced in rabbits. *J. Physiol.
(Lond)*, **232**, 163–79.

Stitt, J. T. (1981). Neurophysiology of fever. *Fed. Proc.*, **40**, 2835–42.

Stitt, J. T. (1985). Evidence for the involvement of the organum vasculosum
laminae terminalis in the febrile response of rabbits and rats. *J. Physiol.
(Lond)*, **368**, 501–11.

Stitt, J. T. (1986). Prostaglandin E as the neural mediator of the febrile
response. *Yale J. Biol. Med.*, **59**, 137–49.

Stitt, J. T. (1991). Differential sensitivity in the sites of fever production by
prostaglandin E_1 within the hypothalamus of the rat. *J. Physiol. (Lond)*,
432, 99–110.

Stitt, J. T. (1993). Central regulation of body temperature. In *Exercise, Heat,
and Thermoregulation*, vol.6. *Perspectives in Exercise Science and Sports
Medicine*, ed. C. V. Gisolfi, D. R. Lamb & E. R. Nadel, pp. 1–39.
Brown & Benchmark, Dubuque, Ia.

Stitt, J. T. & Shimada, S. G. (1991). Site of action of calcium channel
blockers in inhibiting endogenous pyrogen fever in rats. *J. Appl.
Physiol.*, **71**, 956–60.

Stitt, J. T., Shimada, S. G. & Bernheim, H. A. (1984). Microinjection of
zymosan and lipopolysaccharide into the organum vasculosum laminae
terminalis of rats enhances their febrile responsiveness to endogenous
pyrogen. In *Thermal Physiology*, ed. J. R. S. Hales, pp. 555–8. Raven
Press, New York.

Ström, G. (1950). Vasomotor responses to thermal and electrical stimulation of frontal lobe and hypothalamus. *Acta. Physiol. Scand.*, **20**, Suppl.70. 47–111.

Stuart, D. G., Kawamura, Y. & Hemingway, A. (1961). Activation and suppression of shivering during septal and hypothalamic stimulation. *Exptl. Neurol.*, **4**, 485–506.

Stuart, D. G., Kawamura, Y., Hemingway, A. & Price, W. M. (1962). Effects of septal and hypothalamic lesions on shivering. *Exptl. Neurol.*, **5**, 335–47.

Symons, J. A. & Duff, G. W. (1992). Interleukin 1-binding protein: a new soluble cytokine receptor. In *Neuro-immunology of Fever*, ed. T. Bartfai & D. Ottoson, pp. 57–63. Pergamon Press, Oxford.

Székely, M. (1979). Endotoxin fever in the newborn kitten. The role of prostaglandins and monoamines. *Acta Physiol. Acad. Sci. Hung.*, **54**, 265–76.

Székely, M. & Komoromi, I, (1978). Endotoxin and prostoglandin fever of newborn guinea pigs at different ambient temperatures. *Acta Physiol. Acad. Sci. Hung.*, **51**, 293–8.

Székely, M., Sehic, E., Menon, V. & Blatteis, C. M. (1994). Apparent dissociation between lipopolysaccharide-induced intrapreoptic release of prostaglandin E_2 and fever in guinea pigs. In *Temperature Regulation. Recent Physiological and Pharmacological Advances*, ed. A. S. Milton, pp. 65–70. Birkhäuser Verlag, Basel.

Szot, P., Ferris, C. F. & Dorsa, D. M. (1990). [^{3}H] Arginine-vasopressin binding sites in the CNS of the golden hamster. *Neurosci. Lett.*, **119**, 215–18.

Takahashi, Y., Smith, P., Wilkinson, M. J. & Cooper, K. E. (1993). Pyrogen access into the brain. *Proc. Soc. Neurosci. Annual Meeting*, Nov. 7–12. Washington, DC, USA. Abstract. 47.2.

Tangri, K. K., Bhargava, A. K. & Bhargava, K. P. (1974). Interrelation between monoaminergic and cholinergic mechanisms in the hypothalamic centre of rabbits. *Neuropharmacol.*, **13**, 333–46.

Teddy, P. J. (1971). In *Pyrogens and Fever*, ed. G. E. W. Wolstenholme & J. Birch, pp. 124–6. Churchill Livingstone, Edinburgh.

Thornton, S. N., Sirinathsinghji, D. J. & Delaney, C. E. (1987). The effects of a reversible colchicine-induced lesion of the anterior ventral region of the third ventricle in rats. *Brain Res.*, **437**, 339–44.

Tsubokura, S., Watanabe, Y., Ehara, H., Imamura, K., Sugimoto, O., Kagamiyama, H., Yamamoto, S. & Hayaishi, K. (1991). Localization of prostaglandin endoperoxide synthase in neurons and glia in monkey brain. *Brain Res.*, **543**, 15–24.

Van Miert, A. S. J. A. M., Van Duin, C. T. M., Verheijden, J. H. M., Schotman, A. J. H. & Nieuwenhuis, J. (1984). Fever and changes in plasma zinc and iron concentrations in the goat: the role of leucocytic pyrogen. *J. Comp. Pathol.*, **94**, 543–57.

Vane, J. R. (1971). Inhibition of prostaglandin synthesis as a mechanism of action for aspirin-like drugs. *Nature new Biol.*, **231**, 232–5.

Vaughn, L. K., Veale, W. L. & Cooper, K. E. (1979). Fever and survival in a mammal: effects of central antipyresis. In *Thermoregulatory Mechanisms and their Therapeutic Implications*, ed. B. Cox, P. Lomax, A. S. Milton & E. Schönbaum, pp. 115–19. Karger, Basel.

Vaughn, L. K., Veale, W. L. & Cooper, K. E. (1980). Antipyresis: its effect on mortality rate of bacterially infected rabbits. *Brain Res. Bull.*, **5**, 69–73.

Vaughn, L. K., Veale, W. L. & Cooper, K. E. (1981). Effects of antipyresis on bacterial numbers in infected rabbits. *Brain Res. Bull.*, **7**, 175–80.

Veale, W. L. & Cooper, K. E. (1975). Comparison of sites of action of prostaglandin E and leucocyte pyrogen in brain. In *Temperature Regulation and Drug Action*, ed. P. Lomax, E. Schönbaum & J. Jacob, pp. 218–26. Karger, Basel.

Veale, W. L., Kasting, N. W. & Cooper, K. E. (1981). Arginine vasopressin and endogenous antipyresis: evidence and significance. *Fed. Proc.*, **40**, 2750–9.

Villablanca, J. & Myers, R. D. (1965). Fever produced by microinjection of typhoid vaccine into hypothalamus of cats. *Am. J. Physiol.*, **208**, 703–6.

Vogt, M. (1954). The concentration of sympathin in different parts of the central nervous system under normal conditions and after the administration of drugs. *J. Physiol. (Lond)*, **123**, 451–81.

Wallace, S. J. (1976). Neurological and Intellectual deficits: Convulsions with fever viewed as acute indications of life-long developmental deficits. In *Brain Disfunction in Infantile Febrile Convulsions*, ed. M. A. B. Brazier & F. Coceani, pp. 259–77. Raven Press, New York.

Watanabe, Y., Watanabe, Y. & Hayaishi, O. (1988). Quantitative autoradiographic localization of prostaglandin E_2 binding sites in the monkey diencephalon. *J. Neurosci.*, **8**, 2003–10.

Watanabe, Y., Watanabe, Y., Hamada, K., Bommelaer-Boyt, M. C., Dray, F., Kaneko, T., Yumoto, N. & Hayaishi, O. (1989). Distinct localization of prostaglandin D_2, E_2, and $F_{2\alpha}$ binding sites in monkey brain. *Brain Res.*, **478**, 143–8.

Weinberg, E. D. (1984). Iron withholding: a defense against infection and neoplasia. *Physiol. Rev.*, **64**, 65–102.

Weindl, A. & Sofroniew, M. (1985). Neuroanatomical pathways related to vasopressin. In *Current Topics in Neuroendocrinology*, vol.4, ed. D. Ganten & D. Pfaff, pp. 137–95. Springer-Verlag, Berlin.

Weinstein, M. J., Wartz, J. A. & Came, P. E. (1970). Induction of resistance to bacterial infections of mice with PolyI-PolyC. *Nature*, **226**, 170.

Westphal, O. & Luderitz, O. (1954). Chemische Erforschung von Liposacchariden gramnegativer Bakterien. *Angew Chem.*, **66**, 407–17.

Whittet, T. D. (1980). *Pyrogens in the modern setting. The 1980 Todd Lecture*. Printed by Mallinckrodt, Inc., St. Louis, Missouri.

Wilkinson, M. F. & Kasting, N. W. (1990a). Centrally acting vasopressin contributes to endotoxin tolerance. *Amer. J. Physiol.*, **258**, R443–9.

Wilkinson, M. F. & Kasting, N. W. (1990b). Central vasopressin V_1-blockade prevents salicylate but not acetaminophen antipyresis. *J. Appl. Physiol.*, **68**, 1793–8.

Wilkinson, M. F. & Pittman, Q. J. (1994). Alteration of the physiological responses to indomethacin by endotoxin tolerance in the rat: a possible role for central vasopressin. *J. Physiol. (Lond)*. **479**, 441–9.

Wilkinson, M. F., Mathieson, W. B. & Pittman, Q. J. (1993). Interleukin-1β has excitatory effects on neurons of the bed nucleus of the stria terminalis. *Brain Res.*, **625**, 342–6.

Wilkinson, M. F., Horn, T., Kasting, N.W. & Pittman, Q. J. (1994). Interleukin-1β stimulates the bed nucleus of the stria terminalis to release vasopressin into the rat brain. *J. Physiol. (Lond).* (In press.)

Willcox, B. J., Poulin, P., Veale, W. L. & Pittman, Q. J. (1992). Vasopressin-induced motor effects: localization of a sensitive site in the amygdala. *Brain Res.*, **596** (1-2), 58–64.

Williams, J. W., Rudy, T. A., Yaksh, T. L. & Viswanathan, C. T. (1977). An extensive exploration of the rat brain for sites mediating PG-induced hyperthermia. *Brain Res.*, **120**, 251–62.

Withers, P. C. (1978). Bioenergetics of a "primitive" mammal, the Cape Golden Mole. *S. African J. Science.*, **74**, 347–8.

Witt, A. & Wang, S. C. (1968). Temperature sensitive neurons on preoptic/anterior hypothalamic region: actions of pyrogens and acetylsalicylate. *Amer. J. Physiol.*, **215**, 1160–9.

Wolpe, S. D., Sherry, B., Juers, D., Davatelis, G., Yurt, R. W. & Cerami, A. (1989). Identification and characterization of macrophage inflammatory protein 2. *Proc. Natl. Acad. Sci. USA*, **86**, 612–16.

Wolstenholme, G. E. W. & Birch, J. (eds) (1971). *Pyrogens and Fever.* Churchill Livingstone, Edinburgh.

Work, E. (1971). Production, chemistry and properties of bacterial pyrogens and endotoxins. In *Pyrogens and Fever*, ed. G. E. W. Wolstenholme & J. Birch, pp. 23–47. Churchill Livingstone, Edinburgh.

Wunderlich, C. A. (1871). *On the Temperature in Diseases: a Manual of Medical Thermometry*, 2nd edn, pp. 134, 313, translated by W. Bathhurst Woodman. New Sydenham Society, London.

Wurpel, J. N. D., Dundore, R. L., Barbella, Y. R., Balaban, C. D., Keil, L. C. & Severs, W. B. (1986). Barrel rotation evoked by intracerebroventricular vasopressin injections in conscious rats II. Visual/vestibular interactions and efficacy of antiseizure drugs. *Brain Res.*, **365**, 30–41.

Xin, L. & Blatteis, C. M. (1992). A substance P antagonist (ANTISP) inhibits IL-1β effects on neurons in guinea pig preoptic area (PO) tissue slices. *Faseb. J.*, **6** (4), A1199. No.1518.

Yamashita, H., Inenaga, K. & Koizumi, K. (1984). Possible projections from regions of paraventricular and supraoptic nuclei to the spinal cord: electrophysiological studies. *Brain Res.*, **296**, 373–8.

Zeisberger, E. (1989). Antipyretic action of vasopressin in the ventral septal area of the guinea pig's brain. In *Thermoregulation Research and Clinical Applications*, ed. P. Lomax & E. Schönbaum, pp. 65–8. Karger, Basel.

Zeisberger, E. (1991). Peptides and amines as putative factors in endogenous antipyresis. In *New Trends in Autonomic Nervous System Research*, ed. M. Yoshikawa, M. Uono & H. Tanare, pp. 86–9. Elsevier Science Publishers, Amsterdam.

Zeisberger, E., Merker, G. & Blähser, S. (1980). Fever response in the guinea pig before and after parturition and its relationship to the antipyretic reaction of the pregnant sheep. *Brain Res.*, **212**, 392–7.

Zeisberger, E., Merker, G. & Blähser, S. (1983). Changes in activity of vasopressin neurons during fever in the guinea pig. *Neurosci. Lett.* (suppl) 14, S414.

Zeisberger, E., Merker, G., Blähser, S. & Krannig, M. (1986). Role of vasopressin in fever regulation. In *Homeostasis and Thermal Stress*, ed. K. E. Cooper, P. Lomax, E. Schönbaum & W. L. Veale, pp. 62–5. Karger, Basel.

Zeisberger, E., Cooper, K. E., Kluger, M. J., McClellan, J. L. & Roth, J. (1994). Cytokines in endotoxin tolerance. In *Temperature Regulation Advances in Pharmacological Sciences*, ed. A. S. Milton, pp. 17–22. Birkhäuser Verlag, Basel.

Zurovsky, Y., Brain, T., Laburn, H. & Mitchell, D. (1987a). Pyrogens fail to produce fever in the snakes *Psammophis Phillipsii* and *Lamprophis Fuliginosus*. *Comp. Biochem. Physiol.*, **87A**, 911–14.

Zurovsky, Y., Laburn, H. & Mitchell, D. (1987b). Responses of baboons to traditionally pyrogenic agents. *Can. J. Physiol. Pharmacol.*, **65**, 1402–7.

Zurovsky, Y., Mitchell, D. & Laburn, H. (1987c). Pyrogens fail to produce fever in the leopard tortoise Geochelone Pardalis. *Comp. Biochem. Physiol.*, **87A**, 467–9.

Index